All about

Nursing Care

in Oncology

The Complete Guide

ALEXANDRE CAREWELL

Table of Contents

« Each patient is a unique universe, and in Oncology, our mission is to navigate alongside them, transforming obstacles into hope. »

Chapter 1:
INTRODUCTION TO ONCOLOGY

History and development of oncology

Oncology, as we know it today, is the result of centuries of discovery, experimentation and technological advances. But before delving into this rich history, let's go back to the time of ancient civilisations.

It was in ancient Egypt, more than 3,000 years ago, that the first written mention of cancer was found, inscribed on a papyrus. At that time, the disease was still unknown, shrouded in mystery and often associated with superstition. Treatments were rudimentary, based mainly on surgery, with no real understanding of the nature of the disease.

Over the centuries, cancer, from the Latin "crab" - a name given by the Greek physician Hippocrates to describe the way in which the disease spread like a star through the body - has remained an enigma for most doctors and researchers. Galen, another Greek physician, popularised the term "tumour" to describe the abnormal growths seen in certain patients.

It was only in the 19th century, with the advent of the microscope, that scientists began to understand the true cellular nature of cancer. It was then that cancer cells were identified for the first time. This discovery opened the door to a new era of research and understanding.

With the arrival of the 20th century, oncology gradually took shape as a medical speciality. Surgery remained at the heart of treatment, but other modalities, such as radiotherapy, were introduced thanks to the discovery of X-rays. The 1940s saw the emergence of chemotherapy, providing another weapon in the arsenal against cancer.

The modern era of oncology is characterised by a multidisciplinary approach. Advances in genetics and molecular biology have paved the way for targeted therapies, enabling certain cancers to be treated with unprecedented precision. Today, immunotherapy, which uses the patient's own immune system to fight cancer, represents innovation and hope for many patients and healthcare professionals.

The history of oncology is the story of a tireless quest to understand and treat one of the most complex diseases in human history. It is a testament to the triumph of curiosity, perseverance and scientific innovation in the face of medical challenges.

The importance of the nursing role in oncology

Oncology is a demanding and constantly evolving medical speciality, focused on the care of cancer patients. At the heart of this dynamic is the oncology nurse, whose role goes far beyond the administration of care. They play an essential role both in the patient's recovery process and in the mechanics of a close-knit medical team.

To begin with, the complexity of cancer treatment requires a global approach. Cancer patients are often faced with a multiplicity of symptoms, both as a result of the disease itself and the side-effects of treatment. The nurse is often the patient's first point of contact, playing the role of attentive observer, able to detect any change in symptoms, mood or general state of health.

Therapeutic education is also a crucial part of the profession. Patients and their families need to be informed about treatments, their side effects, the steps to take at home, the warning signs to look out for... This is where nurses come in, using their teaching skills and empathy to equip their patients with the knowledge they need to play an active role in their recovery.

The psychological aspect cannot be overlooked either. Faced with a cancer diagnosis, many people experience anxiety, fear and even distress. The oncology nurse, through his or her proximity and availability, offers an attentive ear and emotional support, often becoming a pillar of strength for the patient and his or her family.

As part of the medical team, nurses play a coordinating role. They liaise between doctors, pharmacists, other healthcare professionals and the patient. Their expertise and experience ensure the cohesion and efficiency of the care process.

Finally, with the constant advances in oncology treatments, the nursing profession needs to update its knowledge on a regular basis. Whether through ongoing training, seminars or exchanges with experts, oncology nurses are committed to a constant learning process in order to provide the best possible care.
The oncology nurse is not just an executor of medical orders; he or she is a key player in the care pathway, an ally for the patient, a coordinator for the medical team and an ambassador for innovation in oncology care. Their presence and dedication are major assets in the fight against cancer.

Differences and similarities between oncology and other specialities

By focusing on the prevention, diagnosis, treatment and research of cancers, oncology both differs from and shares certain characteristics with other medical specialities. Here is an exploration of its differences and similarities with other fields:

Differences :
- **Emotional complexity**: Oncology deals with a disease that often evokes fear, uncertainty and, in many cases, a serious prognosis. This can lead to a deeper level of emotional involvement than in other specialities.
- **Interdisciplinarity**: While other specialities work in teams, oncology requires even closer collaboration between various health professionals - surgeons, radiologists, pathologists, pain specialists, psychologists and, of course, oncology nurses.
- **Rapid developments**: Cancer research is progressing at breakneck speed, which means that protocols and treatments are evolving rapidly. This dynamic may be less pronounced in other specialities.
- **Pluripathology**: Oncology patients may suffer from several types of pathology at the same time, particularly as a result of the side effects of treatment.

Similarities :
- **Patient-centred approach**: As in other specialties, oncology aims to provide patient-centred care, taking into account patients' needs, preferences and personal circumstances.
- **Research and innovation**: Although oncology is at the forefront of medical research, other specialities,

such as cardiology and neurology, are also pursuing major innovations.

- **Therapeutic education**: As in oncology, other fields such as diabetes and rheumatology stress the importance of educating patients about their condition, the treatments available and preventive measures.
- **Long-term follow-up**: Many specialities, particularly chronic diseases such as endocrinology or nephrology, require regular, long-term follow-up of patients, as does oncology, especially as part of post-treatment monitoring.

Although oncology has unique characteristics due to the complex nature of cancer, it also shares many common aspects with other medical specialties. These similarities and differences reflect the richness and diversity of medicine, where each field brings its own perspective and expertise to improving the health and well-being of patients.

Chapter 2:
THE BIOLOGY OF CANCER

Understanding the cancer cell

A cancer cell, often referred to in medical literature as a 'malignant cell', is a cell that has undergone a transformation that allows it to multiply uncontrollably and eventually invade other tissues. To understand this transformation, it is essential to explore what differentiates the cancerous cell from its normal counterpart.

- Origin of the cancer cell :
  - All cancer cells derive from a normal cell that has undergone a series of genetic mutations. These mutations can be caused by various factors, such as radiation, certain chemicals, infection by certain viruses, or even hereditary factors.
- Uncontrolled multiplication :
  - Unlike normal cells, which follow a well-regulated life cycle - birth, growth, division and death - cancer cells ignore the signals that normally regulate this cycle. As a result, they divide continuously and in a disorderly fashion.
- Evasion of apoptosis :
  - Apoptosis is the programmed process of cell death. Cancer cells have often developed mechanisms to escape this programmed death, which contributes to their proliferation.

- Angiogenesis :
  - Tumours need nutrients to grow. Cancer cells have the ability to stimulate the formation of new blood vessels to ensure their supply of

oxygen and nutrients, a process known as angiogenesis.
- Invasion and metastasis :
    - Unlike normal cells, which remain in their place of origin, cancer cells can invade neighbouring tissues and travel to other parts of the body via the blood or lymphatic system, creating secondary tumours, or metastases.
- Alteration of the microenvironment :
    - Cancer cells modify their immediate environment, creating a microenvironment that supports their growth and resistance to treatment.
- Evasion of the immune system :
    - Normally, our immune system recognises and destroys abnormal cells. However, cancer cells develop strategies to evade this surveillance, allowing them to proliferate.
- Genomic instability :
    - Cancer cells often exhibit genomic instability, which means that they rapidly accumulate new mutations. This can accelerate their growth, but it can also make them more resistant to treatment.

In conclusion, the cancer cell is a formidable adversary, complex in its biology and its ability to evolve. However, with each discovery about how it works, medical science makes progress towards more targeted and effective treatments, offering the hope of better cancer care in the future.

The different forms of cancer

Cancer is not a single disease, but a group of diseases characterised by the uncontrolled growth of cells. These cells can invade neighbouring tissues and spread to other parts of the body. Cancers are generally named after the organ or cell type where they begin to develop. Here is a non-exhaustive list of the different forms of cancer:

- Cancers of the digestive tract:
    - Oesophageal cancer
    - Stomach cancer
    - Cancer of the colon or rectum (colorectal cancer)
    - Liver cancer
    - Pancreatic cancer
- Cancers of the respiratory system:
    - Lung cancer
    - **Pleural cancer** (often asbestos-related)
- Cancers of the urinary system:
    - Bladder cancer
    - Kidney cancer
- Cancers of the reproductive system:
    - Prostate cancer (in men)
    - Cervical cancer (in women)
    - Endometrial cancer (cancer of the uterus)
    - Ovarian cancer
    - Testicular cancer
- Cancers of the lymphatic and blood systems:
    - **Leukaemia** (cancer of the blood cells)
    - **Lymphoma** (cancer of the lymph nodes)
    - **Myeloma** (cancer of the plasma cells in the bone marrow)
- Cancers of the nervous system:
    - **Gliomas** (cancers of the brain and spinal cord)
- Skin cancer:
    - Basal cell carcinoma and squamous cell carcinoma (non-melanoma cancers)
    - **Melanoma** (a more aggressive cancer linked to melanocytes)

- Cancers of the glands:
  - Thyroid cancer
  - Cancer of the adrenal glands
  - Parathyroid cancer
- Breast cancer:
  - Although breast cancer is mainly diagnosed in women, it can also affect men.
- Head and neck cancers:
- This includes several types of cancer that develop in the mouth, pharynx, larynx, nasal sinuses and thyroid.
- Sarcomas:
- These are cancers of soft tissue (such as muscle, tendon or fat) or bone.
- Paediatric cancers:
- Some cancers are specific to childhood, such as **neuroblastoma**, **retinoblastoma** and **Ewing's sarcoma**.

It is essential to note that each cancer has its own characteristics, treatments and prognosis. What's more, with advances in medicine, new subtypes of cancer are regularly identified, and treatments are becoming increasingly targeted and personalised.

Genetics and risk factors

Our understanding of cancer has progressed enormously in recent decades, thanks in particular to the discovery of the key role played by genetics and its interaction with various risk factors.

1. The genetics of cancer :
- **Somatic mutations**: These mutations appear in a single cell after birth and are generally due to environmental factors or errors that occur when the

cell copies its DNA before dividing. They are not inherited or passed on to descendants.
- **Germline mutations**: These mutations are present from birth and are found in every cell of the body. They are inherited from a parent and can increase the risk of developing certain types of cancer.

2. Cancer susceptibility genes :
- Certain genes, when mutated, significantly increase the risk of developing cancer. The best-known examples are **BRCA1** and **BRCA2**, which are associated with an increased risk of breast and ovarian cancer.

3. Risk factors :
In addition to genetics, many factors can increase the risk of cancer. They fall into several categories:
- Environmental and behavioural factors :
    - **Smoking**: Main risk factor for lung cancer, but also for other types of cancer.
    - **Alcohol**: May increase the risk of several cancers, particularly of the liver, mouth, throat and oesophagus.
    - **Exposure to the sun and UV radiation**: the main causes of skin cancer.
    - **Diet**: An unbalanced diet can increase the risk of certain cancers, while a diet rich in fruit and vegetables can have a protective effect.
- **Infectious factors**: Certain pathogens can increase the risk of cancer.
    - **Human papillomavirus (HPV):** Associated with cervical cancer.
    - **Hepatitis B and C viruses**: associated with liver cancer.
    - **Helicobacter pylori**: May increase the risk of stomach cancer.
- Hormonal and physiological factors :
    - Hormonal imbalances or prolonged exposure to certain hormones can increase the risk of

certain cancers, such as breast or prostate cancer.

- Occupational and environmental factors :
    - Occupational exposure to certain substances, such as asbestos or certain paints, can increase the risk of specific cancers.
    - Air pollution has also been associated with an increased risk of certain cancers.
- Medical history and medication :
    - Certain pre-existing conditions or medical treatments can increase the risk of developing cancer.

Genetics play a crucial role in cancer susceptibility, but the interaction between genetics and various risk factors is complex. Prevention, by recognising and limiting exposure to these factors, remains a key means of reducing the risk of cancer.

Chapter 3:
TECHNICAL ASPECTS

Diagnostic tools and imaging in oncology

One of the most striking advances in oncology is the development of advanced imaging and diagnostic techniques. These tools make it possible not only to detect cancers at an early stage, but also to monitor their progression and guide treatment.

1. Biopsy :
This is one of the most common methods of diagnosing cancer. It involves taking a sample of tissue or cells and examining it under a microscope. Biopsies can be taken by surgery, needle or endoscopy.

2. Endoscopy :
This is a technique that uses a thin, luminous instrument called an endoscope to examine the inside of the body. It is often used to detect cancers of the digestive system, respiratory tract and other internal organs.

3. Medical imaging :
  * **Radiography**: This is one of the oldest imaging techniques. It is often used to detect abnormalities in the lungs, bones and other parts of the body.
  * **Computed tomography (CT)**: This technique uses X-rays to create detailed images of the body from different angles. It is useful for identifying tumours and metastases.
  * **Magnetic resonance imaging (MRI)**: Using a magnetic field and radio waves, MRI provides detailed images of soft tissues, particularly the brain, spinal cord and joints.
  * **Positron emission tomography (PET)**: This measures the metabolic activity of cells and is often

used in combination with CT to locate areas of rapid cancer growth.

- **Ultrasound**: This technique uses sound waves to create images of the inside of the body. It is frequently used to examine the liver, kidneys, pancreas, prostate, breasts and other organs.
- **Mammography**: This is a specific x-ray of the breasts used to screen for breast cancer.

4. Laboratory tests :
Blood tests, such as PSA for prostate cancer or CA-125 for ovarian cancer, can help diagnose and monitor certain cancers.

5. Genetic testing :
These tests are used to identify genetic mutations that could increase the risk of certain cancers. They can also guide treatment by identifying specific mutations present in tumours.

6. Nuclear medicine :
It uses small quantities of radioactive materials to diagnose, assess and treat various types of cancer.

7. Functional and metabolic tests :
They can help to assess organ function and determine how a tumour affects that function.

The choice of diagnostic and imaging tools depends on the type of cancer suspected, its location and other factors. With these advanced techniques, doctors can not only detect and diagnose cancer with greater precision, but also plan more targeted treatments and evaluate their effectiveness.

Treatment techniques: chemotherapy, radiotherapy, immunotherapy

Cancer treatment has evolved considerably over the last century. Chemotherapy, radiotherapy and immunotherapy are the three mainstays of cancer treatment. Each of these modalities has its own distinct mechanisms of action, indications and side effects.

1. Chemotherapy :
Chemotherapy involves drugs that kill cancer cells or stop them multiplying. The drugs can be administered orally or intravenously.

- **Mechanism of action**: Chemotherapeutic agents target rapidly dividing cells, a characteristic feature of cancer cells.
- **Use**: It can be used alone or in combination with other treatments. It may be used to reduce the size of a tumour before surgery or radiotherapy, to treat cancer that has spread, or to reduce the risk of recurrence after surgery.
- **Side effects**: As these drugs also attack other rapidly dividing cells (such as those in the bone marrow, hair follicles and gastrointestinal tract), they can cause side effects such as hair loss, nausea, reduced blood cell counts and other symptoms.

2. Radiotherapy :
Radiotherapy uses high-energy radiation to destroy cancer cells. It can be external (delivered by a machine) or internal (where radioactive sources are placed close to the tumour).
- **Mechanism of action**: Radiation damages the DNA of cells, preventing them from dividing and growing.
- **Use**: Radiotherapy is often used as a complement to surgery or chemotherapy, to treat local tumours or to alleviate certain symptoms.
- **Side effects**: The skin, tissues and exposed organs may be affected, leading to redness, burning, fatigue and other symptoms.

3. Immunotherapy :

Immunotherapy stimulates or modifies the immune system so that it attacks cancer cells more effectively. These treatments have revolutionised the treatment of certain cancers.

- **Mechanism of action**: It aims to "wake up" the immune system or "guide" it to specifically target tumours.
- **Use**: It is currently used to treat many types of cancer, including advanced melanoma, certain cancers of the lung, kidney, bladder and head and neck.
- **Side effects**: These are different from those of chemotherapy and radiotherapy and may include autoimmune reactions, where the immune system mistakenly attacks healthy organs or tissues.

The choice of treatment depends on the type and stage of the cancer, as well as the patient's overall health. The multidisciplinary approach, combining these techniques according to the specific needs of each patient, aims to optimise the effectiveness of the treatment while minimising side effects.

Prevention and safety cytotoxic drugs

Cytotoxic drugs, also known as antineoplastic agents or chemotherapeutics, are used to treat various diseases, including cancer. Because of their mechanism of action on cells, they present risks not only for patients, but also for the healthcare staff who handle them. Ensuring the safety of these medicines is therefore of paramount importance.

1. Risks associated with cytotoxic drugs :

Cytotoxic drugs can affect healthy cells, causing :
- Direct toxicity to cells, tissues or organs.
- Mutagenic, teratogenic or carcinogenic effects.

- Allergic reactions.

Healthcare workers exposed to these drugs may therefore be at risk of :
- Skin or mucous membrane exposure.
- Inhalation of particles.
- Accidental ingestion.

2. Preventive measures :
- **Staff training:** All those handling or administering cytotoxic drugs must be properly trained in their risks and safe procedures.
- **Personal protective equipment (PPE): This** includes nitrile gloves, long-sleeved waterproof gowns, masks and goggles.
- **Aseptic techniques:** It is essential to use aseptic techniques when preparing, handling and administering cytotoxic drugs.
- **Use of secure devices:** This includes laminar flow hoods, biological safety cabinets and closed drug transfer systems.

3. Waste management :
- The waste associated with these medicines, including the PPE used, must be treated as hazardous waste.
- They must be placed in specific, clearly identified containers and disposed of in accordance with local regulations.

4. Accidental exposure protocols :

It is essential to have clearly established protocols for dealing quickly and effectively with any accidental exposure. These include:
- Immediately wash the exposed area.
- Notification of the incident to management.
- Appropriate medical follow-up.

5. Raising patient awareness :

Patients should also be informed of the precautions to be taken at home after receiving cytotoxic drugs, particularly with regard to the disposal of body waste and the handling of bedding and clothing.

Ensuring the safety of cytotoxic drugs is a shared responsibility between manufacturers, pharmacies, healthcare institutions, healthcare professionals and patients. Appropriate training, constant awareness and strict protocols are essential to minimise the risks associated with these powerful drugs.

Chapter 4:
THE ROLE OF THE NURSE

Initial patient assessment

The initial assessment of a patient with suspected or newly diagnosed cancer is a crucial stage in the oncology care pathway. It is at this point that essential information is gathered to guide the diagnosis, prognosis and treatment plan.

1. Anamnesis :
   - **Medical history:** It is important to gather information about the patient's medical history, including previous illnesses, surgical procedures and drug treatments.
   - **History of cancer:** Details of the onset, duration and course of symptoms and any previous treatment.
   - **Family history:** Search for cases of cancer in the family that could indicate a genetic predisposition.
   - **Lifestyle habits:** smoking, alcohol consumption, diet, physical activity, exposure to occupational or environmental carcinogens.

2. Physical examination :
   - **General examination:** Assessment of the patient's general condition, body mass index, energy levels, etc.
   - **Targeted examination:** Focus on specific systems or organs where the patient has symptoms or signs, or where cancer is suspected.

3. Diagnostic assessments :
   - **Imaging:** X-rays, ultrasound, MRI, PET scan, CT scan, etc. These tools can help locate the tumour, determine its size and see if it has spread.

- **Biopsies**: Tissue samples taken for microscopic examination to confirm the presence of cancer cells.
- **Blood tests**: To assess organ function, detect possible metastases or tumour markers.

4. Psychosocial assessment :
- **Emotional state**: looking for signs of distress, anxiety or depression.
- **Social support**: Understanding the patient's support network - family, friends, support groups.
- **Financial and professional assessments**: Understanding the patient's concerns about the cost of care, insurance, impact on work, etc.

5. Functional assessment :
- **Performance Status**: Assessment of the patient's activity level and ability to carry out daily activities. Scales such as ECOG (Eastern Cooperative Oncology Group) or Karnofsky are commonly used.
- **Other functions**: Assessment of ability to swallow, respiratory function, mobility, etc., depending on the location of the cancer.

6. Specialist consultations :
      Depending on the nature and location of the cancer, consultations with specialists such as a surgeon, radiologist, geneticist, nutritionist, etc. may be necessary.

Initial patient assessment in oncology is a comprehensive, multidimensional process that requires a structured, coordinated approach. It provides the essential information needed to draw up an individualised treatment plan and take a holistic approach to cancer, taking into account not only the tumour itself, but also the person as a whole.

Treatment administration

The administration of oncology treatments requires specific expertise. Each treatment modality has its own guidelines, techniques and precautions, making the role of the oncology nurse crucial to the safety and efficacy of the treatment.

1. Chemotherapy :
   * Preparation :
     * Checking medical orders.
     * Preparation in a laminar flow hood to ensure a sterile environment.
     * Use of appropriate personal protective equipment (PPE).
   * Route of administration :
     * Intravenous (IV): via a catheter or port-a-cath.
     * Oral: in pills or liquid.
     * Topical: applied directly to the skin.
     * Intrathecal: directly into the cerebrospinal fluid.
   * Monitoring during administration :
     * Monitoring vital signs.
     * Look for signs of allergic reactions or other adverse reactions.
     * Patient education on what to expect during and after administration.

2. Radiotherapy :
   * Preparation :
     * Initial assessment to determine the scope of treatment.
     * Marking or tattooing of the area to be treated to ensure precision.
   * During treatment :
     * Precise patient positioning.
     * Protection of surrounding healthy tissue.

- Continuous monitoring during exposure to radiation.
- Post-processing advice :
  - Skin care in the treated area.
  - Monitoring of side effects, such as fatigue.

3. Immunotherapy :
- Preparation :
  - Checking medical orders.
  - Often administered by the IV route.
- Monitoring during administration :
  - Monitoring immunological reactions.
  - Patient education on potential side effects.

4. Targeted therapies :
- Preparation and administration :
  - Often administered orally or IV.
  - Specific dosage according to the type of drug and patient.
- Monitoring :
  - Monitoring of side effects specific to each drug.
  - Dosage may be adjusted according to patient tolerance.

5. Patient education :
- Before treatment :
  - Information on the process and what to expect.
  - Discussion of potential side effects.
- After treatment :
  - Advice on managing side effects.
  - Encouraging communication about symptoms and concerns.

6. Specific considerations :
- Staff protection :
  - Appropriate use of PPE.
  - Safe handling of medicines and equipment.

- Patient protection :
    - Ensuring that medicines are administered to the right patient, at the right dosage, by the right route and at the right time.
    - Ongoing assessment of the patient to detect any complications.

The administration of oncology treatments is complex and requires particular attention to precision, safety and monitoring. Oncology nurses play a central role in ensuring that patients receive the highest quality of care while minimising the risks associated with treatment.

Managing side effects

Each patient's experience of cancer and its treatment is unique. Managing side-effects is a crucial part of oncology management to improve patient quality of life and ensure safe administration of treatments. Nurses are often on the front line to educate, monitor and intervene when these side effects occur.

1. Side effects of chemotherapy :
    - Nausea and vomiting:
        - Prescription of antiemetics.
        - Dietary advice: light meals, avoid fatty or spicy foods.
    - Myelosuppression :
        - Monitoring blood counts.
        - Precautions to prevent infection.
        - Administration of growth factors, if necessary.
    - Alopecia (hair loss) :
        - Advice on using scarves, bonnets or wigs.
        - Reassure the patient that this loss is temporary.

- Mucositis (inflammation of the mouth) :
  - Encouraging good oral hygiene.
  - Use of soothing mouthwashes.
  - Tips on avoiding irritating foods.

2. Side effects of radiotherapy :
- Skin reactions :
  - Use of moisturising creams recommended.
  - Avoid exposure to the sun.
  - Avoid tight clothing.
- Fatigue :
  - Encouragement to rest.
  - Planning activities at times of the day when energy levels are at their highest.
- Digestive disorders:
  - Dietary advice: eat small, frequent meals.
  - Administration of anti-nausea medication if necessary.

3. Side effects of immunotherapy :
- Autoimmune reactions :
  - Monitoring of symptoms such as diarrhoea, skin rash or joint pain.
  - Administration of immunosuppressive drugs if necessary.
- Flu-like symptoms :
  - Administration of antipyretics and analgesics.
  - Encouragement to drink plenty of fluids.

4. Psychological management :
- Anxiety and depression:
  - Listening and emotional support.
  - Referral to a psychologist or psychiatrist if necessary.
  - Support groups and complementary therapies.
- Altered body image :
  - Helping patients to express their feelings.
  - Providing resources to manage physical changes.

5. Pain management :
- Regular pain assessment :

- Use of assessment scales.
- Administration of analgesics as prescribed.
- Non-medicinal techniques :
  - Relaxation, meditation and breathing techniques.
  - Physical therapies such as massage or acupuncture.

The side effects of oncology treatments can vary considerably from one patient to another. Effective management requires an individualised approach, proactive education and rapid intervention when symptoms arise. The nurse plays a central role as educator, advocate and support for the patient throughout the treatment journey.

Psychological and relational support

The cancer patient's journey is littered with both physiological and psychological challenges. Carers, particularly nurses, play a key role in providing emotional and relational support, which is as crucial as the medical care itself. The human dimension of oncology is revealed in the complexity of the relationships between carers and patients, and in the weaving of support networks.

1. The importance of communication :
   - Active listening :
     - Be receptive to the patient's concerns.
     - Validate the patient's feelings and emotions without judgement.
   - Therapeutic communication techniques :
     - Ask open-ended questions.
     - Summarise and rephrase to ensure understanding.
     - Use touch, if appropriate, to establish a link.

2. Psychological assessment :
- Identifying signs of distress :
    - Symptoms of anxiety, depression or isolation.
    - Changes in behaviour or mood.
- Use of assessment tools :
    - Pain scales, quality of life questionnaires.

3. Psychological support :
- Referral to professionals :
    - Psychologists, psychiatrists, social workers.
    - Support groups for cancer patients.
- Complementary therapies :
    - Art therapy, music therapy.
    - Meditation, relaxation, breathing techniques.

4. Support at key stages :
- Diagnosis announcement :
    - Support the patient in the initial shock.
    - Providing clear, appropriate information.
- During treatment :
    - Helping to manage the uncertainty and anxiety associated with side effects.
    - Draw up care plans that include psychological needs.
- In remission or at the end of life:
    - Encourage discussion of concerns and hopes.
    - Facilitate conversations about advance directives and end-of-life wishes.

5. The relationship with the family :
- Include the family in discussions:
    - Recognise their support role.
    - Educate people about what to expect and how to help.
- Support groups for relatives :
    - Places where they can express their own fears and concerns.

6. Support for the care team :
- Recognising burn-out:
    - Promoting well-being at work.
    - Encourage moments of decompression.

- Supervision and discussion groups :
    - Spaces where carers can discuss difficult cases.
    - Share experiences and get advice from colleagues.

Cancer affects not only the body, but also the mind. Psychological and relational support is an essential aspect of oncology care. It's a delicate dance between providing a space for expression, active listening, and directing patients towards appropriate interventions. In this dance, the nurse is often on the front line, offering warmth, compassion and expertise every step of the way.

Chapter 5:
COMPLICATION MANAGEMENT

Neutropenia and the risk of infection

Neutropenia, characterised by a reduction in the number of neutrophils (a type of white blood cell) in the blood, is a frequent complication in patients undergoing oncology treatment. This condition exposes patients to an increased risk of potentially serious infections. The role of the nurse is therefore essential in educating, monitoring and intervening rapidly in the event of infectious signs.

1. Understanding neutropenia :
   - Neutrophils and their role :
     - Key players in the immune response to bacterial infections.
     - Actively destroys invading bacteria.
   - Causes of neutropenia in oncology :
     - Side effects of chemotherapy and radiotherapy.
     - Bone marrow diseases, such as leukaemia.
2. Recognising the signs of infection :
   - General symptoms :
     - Fever, chills.
     - Fatigue or malaise.
     - Joint pain or stiffness.
   - Localised symptoms :
     - Redness, heat or pain in a wound.
     - Coughing, shortness of breath or chest pain.
     - Abdominal pain, nausea, vomiting or diarrhoea.
3. Nursing interventions :
   - Patient education :
     - Signs and symptoms of infection to watch out for.
     - Hygiene measures to prevent infections.

- Clinical monitoring :
    - Regular temperature measurement.
    - Monitoring vital signs and symptoms of infection.
    - Blood tests to monitor neutrophil count.
- Interventions in case of fever :
    - Administration of antibiotics in accordance with protocols.
    - Samples taken for bacterial culture.
    - Close monitoring for signs of sepsis.

4. Preventive measures :
- Protective isolation :
    - In the event of severe neutropenia, isolation should be introduced to protect the patient from external infections.
- Rigorous hygiene :
    - Frequent hand washing for both carers and patients.
    - Use of surface disinfectants.
- Nutrition :
    - Advice on foods to avoid to limit the risk of food-borne infections.
    - Encourage a balanced diet to boost the immune system.
- Vaccinations :
    - Update of recommended vaccinations, unless contraindicated.

5. Psychological considerations :
- Anxiety related to neutropenia :
    - Reassure the patient about the measures in place to prevent infections.
    - Offer psychological support to deal with the fear of infection.
- Self-monitoring education :
    - Encourage patients to take responsibility for their own health by monitoring for signs of infection themselves.

Neutropenia is a challenge in the management of oncology patients. Nurses find themselves at the crossroads between education, monitoring and intervention. Effective, proactive management of neutropenia helps to minimise complications and provide patients with the best possible quality of life. The key is anticipation, responsiveness and close collaboration between the patient and the healthcare team.

Metabolic disorders

Metabolic disorders refer to abnormalities in the body's biochemical processes that affect the transformation and use of nutrients. In the context of oncology, these imbalances may arise as a result of the tumour itself, anti-cancer treatments, or as a co-morbidity. Nurses play an essential role in detecting, managing and educating patients about these disorders.

1. Introduction to metabolic disorders :
    * Definition and importance :
    * The basic mechanisms of metabolism.
    * How cancers and their treatments can disrupt these processes.
2. Common metabolic disorders in oncology :
    * Malignant hypercalcaemia :
        * Excessive release of calcium into the blood due to certain tumours.
        * Symptoms: intense thirst, frequent urination, constipation, fatigue, confusion.
    * Tumour lysis syndrome :
        * Rapid destruction of tumour cells, releasing large quantities of substances into the bloodstream.
        * Associated risks: renal failure, cardiac arrhythmias, convulsions.

- Carbohydrate metabolism disorders :
    - Cancers that can alter the body's ability to use glucose, leading to disorders such as diabetes.

3. Diagnosis and monitoring :
- Blood tests :
    - Regular monitoring of electrolyte, glucose and uric acid levels.
    - Early detection of anomalies to avoid complications.
- Clinical evaluation :
    - Identify symptoms suggestive of a metabolic disorder.
    - Continuous patient monitoring.

4. Nursing care and interventions :
- Hydration :
    - Promotes excretion of excess substances.
    - May require intravenous infusion depending on the severity of the condition.
- Medicines :
    - Administration of agents to balance electrolyte levels.
    - For example, bisphosphonates for hypercalcaemia.
- Patient education :
    - Provide information on the signs and symptoms to look out for.
    - The importance of regular monitoring and medical follow-up.

5. Prevention and practical advice :
- Diet :
    - Specific dietary recommendations, for example limiting calcium-rich foods in the event of hypercalcaemia.
- Adherence to treatment :
    - Importance of complying with drug prescriptions to avoid imbalances.

- Physical activity :
    - Stimulates the metabolism and helps regulate a number of bodily processes.

Metabolic disorders are potentially serious complications in oncology. Through careful monitoring, education and early intervention, nurses play a pivotal role in preventing complications and managing affected patients. Working closely with the rest of the medical team, the nurse ensures that the patient receives the best possible care to manage these metabolic challenges.

Pain in oncology

Pain is one of the major concerns of cancer patients. It can result from the tumour itself, from anti-cancer treatments, or from other concomitant conditions. As part of oncology care, it is essential to recognise, assess and treat pain effectively. Nurses, at the heart of patient care, play a central role in this process.

1. Understanding pain in oncology :
    - Types of pain :
        - Nociceptive pain: caused by tissue damage (for example, a tumour pressing against organs or bones).
        - Neuropathic pain: caused by damage to or dysfunction of the nervous system.
        - Mixed pain: combination of the two above.
    - Factors influencing pain :
        - Location and type of cancer.
        - Stage of the disease.
        - Current or previous treatments.
2. Pain assessment :
    - Assessment scales :

- Visual analogue scales, numerical scales, descriptive scales.
- The importance of regular assessment for appropriate care.
  - Pain history :
    - Location, characteristics, duration, triggering or soothing factors.
3. Nursing interventions and management :
  - Medicines :
    - Analgesics: from paracetamol to opioids, depending on the severity of the pain.
    - Co-adjuvant drugs: to treat neuropathic pain or increase the efficacy of analgesics.
  - Non-drug therapies :
    - Relaxation and meditation techniques.
    - Massages, physiotherapy.
    - Acupuncture.
  - Patient education :
    - Information on pain and its treatment.
    - Encourage patients to express their pain and take an active part in managing it.
4. Managing the side effects of pain treatments :
  - Effects of opioids :
    - Constipation, nausea, drowsiness, respiratory depression.
    - The importance of prevention and appropriate care.
  - Monitoring tolerance and dependence :
    - Regular dose adjustments.
    - Assessment of the need for opioid withdrawal or rotation.
5. Psychological aspects of pain :
  - Emotional impact :
    - Pain can cause stress, anxiety and depression.
    - The importance of psychological support.
  - Communication :
    - Create an environment where patients feel safe to talk about their pain.

- Working closely with a multidisciplinary team: oncologists, psychologists, pain specialists.

Pain in oncology is a constant and multidimensional challenge. Holistic management, taking into account physiological, emotional and social aspects, is essential. Nurses, by virtue of their proximity to the patient, are ideally placed to assess, treat and educate patients about their pain, in collaboration with all the healthcare professionals involved in their care.

Complications specific treatments

The fight against cancer is based on a variety of treatments which, while effective, can sometimes lead to severe complications. Oncology nurses must be able to recognise these complications at an early stage, intervene where possible and refer patients to the appropriate specialists. They are also responsible for the therapeutic education of patients, informing them of the risks and warning signs.

1. Chemotherapy :
   - Mucositis:
     - Inflammation and ulceration of mucous membranes, particularly oral.
     - Advice on oral hygiene, soft diet, pain management.
   - Peripheral neuropathies :
     - Sensory, motor or autonomic disorders.
     - Monitoring, prevention (avoiding the cold, for example) and appropriate medication.
   - Myelosuppression :
     - Decreased production of blood cells.
     - Risks of infection, anaemia and bleeding.

2. Radiotherapy :
- Skin reactions :
    - Erythema, desquamation, burns.
    - Local care, moisturising creams, UV protection.
- Fatigue :
    - Accumulative, sometimes persisting after treatment.
    - Advice on making everyday life more comfortable and encouraging adapted physical activity.
- Swallowing problems (during cervical irradiation) :
    - Pain, false routes.
    - Adapted diet, postures, possible rehabilitation.

3. Immunotherapy :
- Autoimmune reactions :
    - Skin, digestive and respiratory disorders, etc.
    - Monitoring of signs, immunosuppressive treatment if necessary.
- Cytokine release syndrome :
    - Fever, fatigue, heart problems.
    - Hospitalisation, drug treatments.

4. Hormone therapy :
- Mood disorders :
    - Depression, irritability.
    - Psychological support, appropriate treatment if necessary.
- Hot flushes :
    - Particularly with anti-estrogenic treatments.
    - Adaptation advice, symptomatic treatments.
- Osteoporosis :
    - Fragility of bones.
    - Calcium and vitamin D supplementation, bisphosphonates.

5. Targeted therapies :
- Skin toxicities :
    - Rashes, dryness, pruritus.
    - Dermatological care, dose adjustment.

- Liver disorders :
    - Increased liver enzymes, hepatitis.
    - Biological monitoring, symptomatic treatment.

The range of oncology treatments is vast, and there are many potential complications. Nurses, on the front line, need to be aware of these complications in order to act and educate effectively. Interdisciplinary management, combined with constant vigilance, optimises patient comfort and safety throughout the course of treatment.

Chapter 6:
END OF LIFE AND PALLIATIVE CARE

Holistic approach to the patient in terminal phase

Caring for a terminally ill patient is one of the most delicate, but also one of the most essential, challenges in the field of oncology. Beyond the physical symptoms, it is the whole person - their emotions, beliefs, relationships and needs - that is at the heart of the concerns. The holistic approach seeks to encompass all these aspects, recognising that each patient is unique and so is their experience of illness and the end of life.

In this context, it is no longer just a question of recovery, but of quality of life, dignity and comfort. Every gesture, every word, every decision must be tinged with respect, empathy and kindness. The nurse plays a pivotal role here, often the first point of contact, the one who observes, reassures and supports.

Pain, which is omnipresent, is not just physical. It is also emotional, psychological, even spiritual. It evokes fear, loss and anticipated mourning. Pain management is multi-dimensional: from analgesics to complementary therapies and psychological and spiritual support.

The social and relational needs of patients are not left out. Families and friends are all profoundly affected by the patient's approach to the end of life. They need to be heard, supported and guided. Discussions about advance directives and end-of-life wishes are approached with sensitivity, but also with clarity, enabling patients and their families to prepare, understand and accept.

The spiritual aspect, too often neglected, is of crucial importance to many patients. Whether it's religious rituals, meditation, or simply deep conversations, there needs to be a space for these existential questions, for this search for meaning that often accompanies the terminal phase.

Finally, death itself. An intimate moment, sacred for some, it must be surrounded by gentleness and respect. The environment, the comfort care, the discreet but benevolent presence of the nursing team, all contribute to making this moment a peaceful passage.

The holistic approach to the terminally ill patient is not just a series of actions or protocols. It is a philosophy, a posture, that places the patient and his or her totality at the centre of our concerns, recognising the richness and complexity, but also the fragility, of human life.

Pain management in the terminal phase

Pain in the terminal phase is one of the major concerns of carers and families. It can be omnipresent, changeable, sometimes elusive, but always dreaded. This pain is not simply physical; it also encompasses emotional, psychological and spiritual dimensions. Holistic pain management is essential to ensure that patients enjoy quality of life and dignity right up to the end.

At a **physiological** level, pain may be due to the progression of the disease, the side effects of treatment or other concomitant pathologies. To assess pain, it is essential to use appropriate pain scales and to understand its nature (nociceptive, neuropathic), intensity and location. Painkillers, from the simplest to strong opioids such as morphine, are the mainstay of this treatment. They must be administered according to the principle of escalation, starting with the least potent, while rapidly adapting doses to achieve optimum relief.

But in addition to drugs, other approaches have been shown to be effective. **Physiotherapy**, **thermal therapy** (hot or cold), certain **nerve stimulation** techniques and **acupuncture** can all be used. It is also possible to consider **surgical intervention** to block certain stubborn pains.

Emotionally and psychologically, pain is closely linked to fear, anxiety and the anticipated loss of self. It is therefore crucial to discuss these aspects with the patient. Psychological support, whether provided by a psychologist, a psychiatrist or even the nursing team, is fundamental. Anxiolytics and antidepressants can also help.

The **spiritual** dimension of pain is particularly important in the terminal phase. For some patients, pain can be experienced as a punishment, or be linked to deep existential questions. Spiritual support, whether provided by a chaplain, imam, rabbi, Buddhist monk or any other spiritual figure, can help patients to find meaning and peace in their pain.

Lastly, communication is the cornerstone of this care. Every patient is unique, and so is every pain. Listening, observing, adjusting treatments and reassuring are all part of the daily routine that ensures real relief.

Managing pain in the terminal phase is an art, requiring both technical skills and profound humanity. The ultimate aim is to enable patients to live out their final moments as serenely as possible, surrounded by their loved ones and free from suffering.

Support for family and friends

When faced with illness, it's not just the patient who is affected, but a whole circle of loved ones who gravitate around them, sharing their worries, hopes and pain. Family and friends are all affected in profound and different ways. They play a central role in supporting the patient, but they in turn are looking for support and understanding. Their psychological and emotional well-being is intrinsically linked to the patient's quality of life.

When the diagnosis is announced, the shock is often brutal. The news of a serious illness such as cancer generates a multitude of emotions: denial, anger, sadness, fear. It is essential that the medical team takes the time to include the family in these initial discussions, answering questions, clarifying doubts and offering a listening ear.

As the disease progresses, those close to them are faced with a variety of challenges. Uncertainty about the outcome, long hours in hospital, care at home and feelings of helplessness all generate considerable stress. Healthcare staff need to be trained to recognise these signs of distress and direct families to the appropriate resources: psychologists, social workers, support groups.

Support groups are particularly beneficial. They offer a safe space where families can share their experiences, fears and hopes with others who are going through similar ordeals. The feeling that they are not alone in this battle is often a source of comfort.

For families with children, the situation becomes even more complex. How do you talk to a child about their illness? How do you explain their parent's absence from home? How do you reassure them? Specialists trained in child psychology can intervene to help parents navigate these troubled waters, ensuring the child's emotional well-being.

When the disease progresses to an advanced or terminal phase, support for the family becomes even more crucial. Discussions about end-of-life care, advance directives and palliative care support need to be approached with sensitivity. After the death, the work of mourning begins, a path strewn with pitfalls. Support must continue, whether through bereavement therapies, support groups or simply a sympathetic ear.

Illness affects not just the patient, but the whole community around them. Support for family and friends is an essential part of oncology care, a responsibility shared by the entire medical team. Caring for family and friends also means caring for the patient, because their well-being is inextricably linked.

Chapter 7:
THE EMOTIONAL DIMENSION

Coping with stress and burnout

Working in oncology is undoubtedly one of the most demanding medical specialities, both physically and emotionally. Confronted daily with suffering and death, but also with hope and healing, oncology healthcare professionals are often on an emotional frontline. The accumulated burden can lead to chronic stress and, ultimately, burnout. Understanding and recognising these phenomena is crucial to ensuring the well-being of carers and, by extension, the quality of care offered to patients.

Stress in oncology can have many causes: the daily confrontation with death, ethical dilemmas, the pressure to make crucial decisions, the frenetic pace of certain units, or managing relationships with patients and their families. When this stress is persistent and poorly managed, it can lead to **burnout**. Burnout manifests itself as intense fatigue, loss of interest in work, reduced empathy and a deterioration in interpersonal relationships.

So how do we meet these challenges?
- **Recognition and awareness**: The first step towards a solution is often to recognise the problem. Hospitals and clinics need to make their teams aware of the signs of stress and burnout and promote a culture where it is acceptable to talk about difficulties.
- **Stress management training**: Workshops and seminars on stress management techniques such as meditation, mindfulness and relaxation techniques can be a great help.
- **Supervision and psychological support**: Setting up regular supervision sessions where carers can

discuss their difficult cases, their emotions and their reactions, can help to defuse many stressful situations.

- **Work-life balance**: Encouraging teams to take time for themselves, to disconnect, to spend time with their families, to engage in relaxing or sporting activities, is crucial to recharging the batteries.
- **Peer support groups**: Creating spaces where professionals can share their experiences, challenges and successes can provide a valuable emotional outlet.
- **Review work organisation**: Excessive workloads, erratic working hours and lack of breaks can contribute to burnout. So it's essential to regularly assess how your work is organised and make any necessary adjustments.
- **Ongoing training**: Regularly updating your knowledge and skills can boost your sense of competence and efficiency, thereby reducing stress.

Dealing with stress and burnout is not a one-off event, but a long-term commitment that requires the involvement of all players in the healthcare system. By taking care of their carers, healthcare establishments guarantee the quality and humanity of the care offered to their patients.

The nurse-patient relationship: building trust

In the complex and often destabilising world of medicine, and particularly in oncology, the relationship between nurse and patient plays a cardinal role. It is a therapeutic alliance in which the nurse, through his or her expertise and empathy, guides, reassures and supports the patient through the meanders of diagnosis, treatment and follow-up. Establishing trust is therefore essential to the success of this relationship.

Trust is not automatic; it has to be built, nurtured and maintained. For patients, illness is often synonymous with vulnerability, anxiety and sometimes even isolation. In this context, the nurse is a pillar of trust, a partner of choice, a companion.

1. Active listening: The first step in building trust is to really listen. The nurse must be available and attentive to what the patient is saying, whether verbally or non-verbally. This active listening helps to identify the patient's concerns, fears and hopes.

2. Clear and transparent communication : To build solid trust, nurses must be able to provide information that is accurate, understandable and tailored to the patient's needs. This sometimes involves simplifying complex medical jargon or explaining the same procedure several times until the patient feels secure.

3. Empathy: Empathy is the ability to put yourself in another person's shoes, to feel and understand what they are going through. This is an essential trait for nurses. It enables them to establish an emotional bond, a closeness that reassures and soothes.

4. Consistency: Trust is also nurtured by consistency in the relationship. Regular monitoring, predictable attitudes and constant availability reinforce the patient's feeling of security.

5. Honesty: If the nurse does not know how to answer a question or if a situation is uncertain, it is essential to be honest and to say so. This avoids creating false expectations and reinforces credibility.

6. Confidentiality: Respecting the confidentiality of patient information is not only a legal and ethical obligation, it is also a guarantee of trust. Patients need to know that their data, confidences and privacy are protected.

7. Commitment: Showing patients that you are genuinely committed to their well-being, their recovery and their support means reassuring them that they are not alone in this ordeal.

In the emotional storm that illness can represent, the nurse-patient relationship is a beacon, a reassuring point of reference. Establishing and maintaining this trust is an art, an essential skill to guarantee not only the quality of care, but also the well-being and serenity of the patient. In oncology, this trust can make all the difference, offering hope and comfort at the most difficult of times.

The importance of teamwork

The multidimensional nature of oncology requires a collaborative approach. Cancer patients are not only faced with a physical illness; they are also confronted with a whirlwind of emotions, decisions to be made and upheavals in their daily lives. Cancer treatment is not the task of a single professional, but that of a close-knit, committed and complementary team.

1. Comprehensive care: Cancer affects the body on several levels. There is, of course, the tumour itself, but also the side-effects of treatment, the emotional and psychological repercussions, and the social and family impacts. A team made up of oncologists, nurses, psychologists, dieticians, social workers and other specialists provides a holistic approach to all these aspects.

2. Complementary skills: Each member of the team brings unique expertise. The oncologist can determine the best treatment plan, the nurse supports and reassures the patient on a daily basis, the psychologist helps manage stress and emotions, and the dietician provides advice on managing treatment-related eating disorders. This synergy ensures that patients benefit from the best knowledge and skills available.

3. Cohesive communication: In a close-knit team, information flows smoothly and efficiently. This ensures that each professional has access to the most recent and relevant data concerning the patient. This is essential to avoid errors and duplication and to guarantee continuity of care.

4. Emotional and professional support: Working in oncology is rewarding, but it's also hard work. There are many emotional challenges. Being part of a team means having colleagues you can count on, with whom you can share your concerns, successes and doubts. This solidarity is a bulwark against burnout.

5. Intellectual stimulation: Medicine is a constantly evolving field. In a team, members can discuss the latest research, share their experiences and learn from each other. It's fertile ground for innovation and excellence.

6. Personalised care: Thanks to a multidisciplinary team, it is possible to tailor care to the individual needs of each patient. Everyone is unique, and the collaborative approach means that we can respond to each person's specific needs.

Teamwork in oncology is not just an option, it's a necessity. It is at the heart of optimal patient care, ensuring that every aspect of the patient's illness is addressed with skill, compassion and efficiency. In this human and medical adventure, professional solidarity is an invaluable strength, for both carers and patients.

Chapter 8:
CASE STUDIES

Case 1: Lymphoma and complications

Lymphoma is a cancer that develops from lymphocytes, a type of white blood cell that is essential for the proper functioning of our immune system. As with all cancers, the treatment of lymphoma requires a global approach, because in addition to the disease itself, patients may encounter various complications, linked either to the disease or to the treatments.

1. Complications associated with the disease :
   - **Tumour syndrome:** In some cases, cancer cells break down rapidly, releasing substances into the bloodstream that can cause kidney problems or heart problems.
   - **Spinal cord compression:** The growth of a tumour mass can compress the spinal cord, causing pain, weakness or even paralysis.
   - **Weakened immune system:** Because lymphoma affects the immune system, patients are often more susceptible to infections.
   - **Superior vena cava syndrome:** Compression or obstruction of the superior vena cava by a tumour can cause swelling of the face, neck, arms and upper chest.
   - **Fluid build-up:** Some lymphomas can cause fluid build-up around the heart (pericarditis) or lungs (pleurisy).

2. Treatment-related complications :
   - **Neutropenia:** Chemotherapy can lead to a reduction in white blood cells, increasing the risk of infections.

- **Anaemia:** A reduction in red blood cells can cause fatigue, paleness and shortness of breath.
- **Thrombocytopenia:** A reduction in blood platelets may cause bleeding or bruising.
- **Cardiac toxicity:** Some medicines can affect the heart, so it is essential to monitor heart function regularly during treatment.
- **Peripheral neuropathy:** Some treatments can affect the nerves, causing tingling, pins and needles or pain.
- **Tumour lysis syndrome: This is a** medical emergency caused by the rapid release of tumour cells into the bloodstream after the start of treatment.
- **Infertility:** Chemotherapy and radiotherapy can affect fertility.
- **Second cancers:** Although rare, treatment for lymphoma can increase the risk of developing another type of cancer in the future.

The management of lymphoma requires rigorous medical monitoring to detect and treat these complications quickly. It can be a challenging journey, but with a holistic approach that takes into account both the disease and the patient's overall well-being, many challenges can be overcome. Research also continues to advance treatments, reducing side effects and improving survival rates.

Case 2: Carcinoma of the breast and post-operative reconstruction

Breast cancer is one of the most common cancers in women. The diagnosis and treatment of breast cancer can have profound repercussions, both physically and emotionally. For many women, part of the healing process after a mastectomy (removal of the breast) or conservative surgery is breast reconstruction. This reconstruction plays an essential role in physical and psychological rehabilitation.

1. Why opt for breast reconstruction?
   - **Restoration of body image:** For some women, breast reconstruction helps to restore self-confidence and overcome the trauma associated with the loss of a breast.
   - **Symmetry:** If only one breast has been affected by cancer, reconstruction can help to restore symmetry between the two breasts.
   - **Personal choice:** Every woman is different. Some may choose not to undergo reconstruction or to wear an external breast prosthesis. The decision whether or not to reconstruct the breast is a deeply personal one.

2. Breast reconstruction options :
   - **Reconstruction by prosthesis:** This method uses silicone or saline implants to reshape the breast. This is one of the most common techniques.
   - **Autologous reconstruction:** Also known as "body tissue reconstruction", this uses tissue from other parts of the body, such as the abdomen, thigh or back, to create a new breast.
   - **Combined reconstruction:** This approach combines the use of implants and autologous tissue.
   - **Nipple and areola reconstruction:** After reconstructing the breast, some women also choose to reconstruct the nipple and areola for a more natural appearance.

3. Moments conducive to reconstruction :
   - **Immediate reconstruction:** This is done at the same time as the mastectomy. Only one operation is required, which may be less traumatic for some women.

- **Delayed reconstruction:** This is carried out after the mastectomy, often after other treatments such as chemotherapy or radiotherapy.
4. What you need to know before taking the plunge :
  - **Variable results:** The results of reconstruction vary from woman to woman. It is important to discuss expectations and possible outcomes with your surgeon.
  - **Possible complications:** As with any surgery, there are risks associated with breast reconstruction, such as infection, implant complications or scarring.
  - **Sensitivity: The** sensitivity of the reconstructed breast may differ from that of the original breast.
  - **Medical follow-up:** Even after reconstruction, it is crucial to continue regular check-ups to ensure that the cancer does not return.

The decision to undergo breast reconstruction after breast carcinoma is an intimate and individual journey. With today's medical advances, women have more options than ever to regain a sense of fulfilment and well-being after a breast cancer diagnosis.

Case 3: Sarcoma:
a multidisciplinary challenge

Sarcomas are a heterogeneous group of cancers that develop in connective tissues such as bone, muscle, tendon, cartilage and fat. Because of their rarity and diversity, their management requires a multidisciplinary approach to ensure the best possible treatment and follow-up.

1. Characteristics of sarcoma :
  - **Diversity:** Sarcomas can occur in any part of the body, and there are over 70 histological subtypes.

This presents specific diagnostic and therapeutic challenges.

- **Rare:** Sarcomas account for only around 1% of all cancers in adults, but they are more common in children.
- **Variable aggressiveness:** Not all sarcomas are aggressive. Some may grow slowly and remain localised, while others are very aggressive and metastatic.

2. The importance of a multidisciplinary approach :

- **Accurate diagnosis:** An accurate diagnosis is crucial in determining the type and stage of the sarcoma. This requires close collaboration between radiologists, pathologists and oncologists.
- **Treatment planning :** Treatment options may include surgery, chemotherapy, radiotherapy or a combination of these methods. A committee of specialists, including surgeons, medical oncologists and radiotherapists, often meets to draw up a plan tailored to each patient.
- **Reconstruction:** In cases where a sarcoma requires major surgery, plastic surgeons may be called in for reconstruction, in order to preserve function and appearance as much as possible.

3. The crucial role of monitoring :

- **Early detection of recurrence:** Sarcomas, particularly aggressive forms, can recur. Regular follow-up with imaging examinations is essential for early detection of any recurrence.
- **Rehabilitation:** Because of the potential impact on function (for example, if the sarcoma is located near a major joint or muscle), patients may need physiotherapy or other forms of rehabilitation.
- **Psychological support:** The often aggressive nature of sarcoma, combined with the complexity of its treatment, can have psychological repercussions. Psychological support or counselling services are

often essential to help patients navigate through these challenges.

4. Research and development :

Given the rarity of sarcomas, collaborative research is crucial. International networks and consortia are focusing on developing new treatments and understanding the biology of sarcomas.

The management of sarcomas symbolises the importance of a multidisciplinary approach to oncology. From accurate diagnosis to treatment planning and post-treatment follow-up, each stage requires the collaboration of dedicated specialists to offer patients the best possible chance of success and quality of life.

Chapter 9:
COMMUNICATION IN ONCOLOGY

The skills you need
for effective communication

In the vast world of human interaction, communication is the keystone. It is through communication that we express our needs, ideas, feelings and intentions. So, for communication to be truly effective, it is imperative to have a set of skills that go far beyond the simple transmission of information. Let's take a look at the essential skills you need to master for truly effective communication.

1. Active listening :
Even before speaking, it is crucial to learn how to listen. Active listening requires total attention to the speaker, avoiding interruptions while giving signs of engagement, such as nodding or eye contact.

2. Clarity and conciseness :
Simplicity is often the best way to avoid misunderstandings. It's important to formulate your thoughts clearly and concisely, avoiding unnecessary jargon or superfluous details.

3. Adaptability :
Not all people are the same. Knowing how to adapt your language, tone and approach to suit your audience means that your message is better received.

4. Empathy :
The ability to put oneself in the other person's shoes is central. This enables us not only to understand the other person's point of view, but also to respond appropriately to their feelings or concerns.

5. Mastering non-verbal language :

Most of our communication is non-verbal. Facial expressions, posture, tone of voice and gestures can all convey messages, sometimes more powerfully than words themselves.

6. Managing emotions :

It's essential to know how to manage your emotions, especially in conflict situations. Keeping calm, avoiding defensiveness and acknowledging your own feelings are crucial steps.

7. Formulating questions :

Asking the right questions - at the right time - can help to clarify ambiguities, deepen a discussion or encourage the other person to express themselves further.

8. Constructive feedback :

Giving and receiving feedback is an essential skill. It is important to know how to provide feedback constructively, focusing on specific points and avoiding personal attacks.

9. Assertiveness :

Expressing your needs, feelings or opinions respectfully but clearly is an essential skill. This avoids misunderstandings and builds mutual trust.

10. Patience :

Patience is often underestimated, but it is fundamental. Waiting for the right moment to speak, giving the other person time to express themselves or thinking before responding are all practices that promote harmonious communication.

By developing and refining these skills, you can build more rewarding and satisfying relationships, both professionally and personally. In a world where misinformation and misunderstandings are commonplace, effective communication is more valuable than ever.

Obstacles of good communication

Communication is a skill which, although natural, can often be hampered by various obstacles. These barriers can make the transmission of information difficult or even impossible. They can also lead to misunderstandings, frustration and conflict. Identifying these barriers is the first step towards smoother, more effective communication. Here is an overview of the most common barriers to good communication:

1. Environmental distractions :
Loud noises, a chaotic environment or even visual distractions can hamper concentration, making it difficult to listen and understand.

2. Incoherent non-verbal language :
Body language, facial expressions and tone of voice can convey a different message from the words used, creating confusion.

3. Cultural barriers :
Cultural differences can influence the way messages are perceived and interpreted. Gestures or expressions that are common in one culture may be misunderstood or even offensive in another.

4. Strong emotions :
Anger, sadness, excitement or stress can cloud the message. When we are overwhelmed by emotions, we may find it difficult to listen or express ourselves clearly.

5. Prejudice and stereotypes :
Having preconceived ideas or stereotypes about a person or group can affect the way we receive and interpret their messages.

6. Poor listening :
Listening passively, without really paying attention, is a major obstacle to effective communication.

7. Information overload :

Being overwhelmed by too much information at once can make it difficult to digest and retain the message.

8. Excessive use of jargon :

Relying on technical or domain-specific terms without explaining them can exclude those who are unfamiliar with the subject.

9. Physical barriers :

Hearing, vision or other disabilities can make communication more difficult.

10. Assumptions and jumping to conclusions :

Assuming that you know what the other person is thinking or feeling without checking can lead to misunderstandings.

11. Lack of assertiveness :

Not expressing your own needs, feelings or opinions can prevent open and honest communication.

12. Closed-mindedness :

Not being open to new ideas or perspectives can prevent genuine understanding and exchange of information.

13. Language problems :

Communication between people who speak different languages or dialects can present obvious challenges.

By recognising these barriers and being aware of their influence, we can work to overcome them, by adapting our communication style and developing skills to facilitate more harmonious interaction. Every effort to overcome these barriers brings us closer to more transparent, authentic and effective communication.

Difficult discussions:
announce a diagnosis,
a repeat offence, the end of life...

Passing on news, especially when it is upsetting or unexpected, is one of the most sensitive responsibilities of healthcare staff. These discussions are particularly important in oncology, where the news can radically change the lives of patients and their families. Navigating these exchanges with compassion, honesty and sensitivity is essential. Here's a look at how to approach these difficult discussions.

1. Preparing for the conversation :
It is essential to prepare yourself mentally and emotionally for these exchanges. This involves not only understanding all the medical details, but also connecting with your own sense of empathy and compassion.

2. Creating the right environment :
Choose a place that is calm, private and free from distractions. Make sure the patient is comfortable and has plenty of time to digest the information.

3. Presence and active listening :
The importance of being fully present and attentive cannot be underestimated. Patients need to feel that they are the priority, that their feelings, questions and concerns will be heard.

4. Communicate clearly and honestly :
It's crucial to be direct, but also sensitive. Use clear language, avoid complicated medical jargon and make sure the patient and family understand the information.

5. Let the patient express his or her emotions:
It is normal for patients to experience a range of emotions. Whether it's shock, sadness, anger or confusion, allow them to express themselves without judgement.

6. Offer support :
After delivering the news, suggest resources to help the patient manage the situation. This could include referrals to support groups, therapists or other specialists.

7. Involving the family :
With the patient's permission, it may be beneficial to include family members in these discussions. They can offer valuable support and may also have their own questions or concerns.

8. Provide options where possible:
If there are treatment options or other decisions to be made, present them in a clear and understandable way. Give patients the time and space they need to reflect on these choices.

9. Confirm understanding :
After sharing the news, check that the patient has understood the information. Encourage them to ask questions and express their concerns.

10. Follow up :
It may take some time for the news to sink in. Schedule another appointment or follow-up call to discuss any further questions or concerns.

11. Take care of yourself:
As a healthcare professional, it is essential to recognise the emotional impact these conversations may have on you. Seek support if necessary, whether through colleagues, supervision or counselling.

It is essential to approach these discussions with compassion, patience and empathy. Even if the news is difficult, respect and understanding can make this painful process easier for the patient and their family.

Chapter 10:
ETHICAL ASPECTS IN ONCOLOGY

Decision-making in complex situations

In the medical field, particularly in oncology, professionals are often faced with complex decisions that have major implications for patients' lives. These decisions may involve treatment choices, ethical dilemmas or situations where the outcome is uncertain. Navigating these turbulent waters requires a combination of technical, emotional and ethical skills.

1. Recognising complexity :
The first step is to recognise that the situation is complex. This means accepting that there may not be a "right" answer and that each decision can have both positive and negative consequences.

2. Gathering information :
Before making a decision, it is crucial to gather all the relevant information. This includes medical details, patient history, patient and family preferences and available resources.

3. Evaluating the options :
Once all the information is gathered, consider the different options available. Each option should be assessed in terms of its benefits, risks, costs and potential long-term consequences.

4. Consult and collaborate :
Engage with other healthcare professionals, colleagues, multidisciplinary teams and, where appropriate, the patient's relatives. These consultations may bring new perspectives or additional information that could influence the decision.

5. Integrating patient preferences and values :
In medicine, the patient is at the centre of care. It is

therefore essential to incorporate their preferences, values and wishes into the decision-making process.

6. Ethical reflection :

Some situations require careful reflection on the ethical implications. These considerations may include the patient's well-being, respect for autonomy, justice and non-harm.

7. Clear communication :

It is essential to communicate the decision, and the reasoning behind it, in a clear and understandable way to the patient and family. This helps to build trust and facilitates acceptance of the decision.

8. Ongoing evaluation :

Once a decision has been made, it is crucial to continually evaluate the situation. Circumstances may change, new information may emerge, and re-evaluation may be necessary.

9. Accept uncertainty :

In oncology, as in other areas of medicine, there can be inherent uncertainty. Accepting this uncertainty and being transparent about it with the patient is crucial.

10. Emotional support:

Complex decisions can have an emotional impact on both the healthcare professional and the patient. Be sure to seek emotional support where necessary and offer this support to the patient and their family.

11. Self-reflection:

Take time to reflect on complex decisions, learn from each situation and continually improve your decision-making skills.

Decision-making in complex situations is a skill that develops with time, experience and reflection. It requires a combination of rational analysis, intuition, compassion and respect for the patient's dignity and autonomy.

Common ethical dilemmas

In the medical field, and particularly in oncology, ethical dilemmas are omnipresent. These challenges can arise at any time, testing the values, convictions and professional conscience of carers. Here is an overview of the most commonly encountered ethical dilemmas and the considerations that underlie them.

1. Autonomy vs. charity :
   - **Issue:** A patient refuses a treatment which, according to the medical team, is in his best interests.
   - **Considerations:** Respecting the patient's right to self-determination while seeking to act for his or her well-being.
2. Full information vs. hope :
   - **Issue:** To what extent should a patient be informed of a poor prognosis without giving up hope?
   - **Considerations:** Balance between transparency and the desire to protect patient morale.
3. Life extension vs. quality of life :
   - **Issue:** Should we continue with invasive treatments that could prolong life but reduce its quality?
   - **Considerations:** Weigh up the benefits against the potential suffering.
4. Limited resources vs. optimal care :
   - **Problem:** How do you decide how to allocate limited resources, such as an expensive drug or limited access to an imaging machine?
   - **Considerations:** Balance between equity, utility and need.
5. Respect for cultural values vs. medical standards :
   - **Issue: How** should we react when a patient's cultural or religious beliefs conflict with medical recommendations?
   - **Considerations:** Recognising the importance of individual values while adhering to standards of care.

6. Confidentiality vs. protection of others :
   - **Issue:** Should confidentiality be broken if a patient poses a risk to themselves or others?
   - **Considerations :** Weighing the right to privacy against the duty to protect.
7. End-of-life decisions :
   - **Issue:** When, how and under what conditions should life-sustaining care be stopped or comfort measures only be implemented?
   - **Considerations:** Respect the patient's wishes, quality of life and the opinions of family members and the medical team.
8. Clinical research vs. patient care :
   - **Issue:** How can the needs of medical research be balanced with the individual interests of the patient when taking part in a clinical trial?
   - **Considerations:** Ensure full information, informed consent and protect patient rights.
9. The challenges of informed consent :
   - **Issue:** How can we ensure that patients fully understand the implications, risks and benefits of a treatment or procedure?
   - **Considerations:** Provide clear information, allow time for questions, and assess the patient's decision-making capacity.

Each of these dilemmas requires a thoughtful approach, balancing ethical principles, patient needs and medical realities. Engaging in open, honest and compassionate discussions is essential to navigating these delicate waters.

Informed consent and the patient's ability

Informed consent is a cornerstone of ethical, patient-centred medical practice. It recognises and respects patient autonomy by enabling patients to make informed decisions about their health. However, the informed consent process is intrinsically linked to the patient's ability to understand, assess and decide. It is a delicate dance between respecting patients' rights and ensuring their protection.

1. Foundations of informed consent :
Informed consent is based on the principle that each individual has the right to decide what is done to them medically. For consent to be truly "informed", the patient must :
- Understand the information provided.
- Evaluate the options available.
- Decide freely, without constraint or undue influence.

2. Informed consent process :
- **Information:** The healthcare professional must provide the patient with all relevant information concerning the diagnosis, prognosis, treatment options, risks, benefits and alternatives.
- **Understanding:** It is crucial to ensure that the patient has understood all this information. This may involve explaining complex concepts in simple, accessible language.
- **Decision:** Once informed, patients make a choice based on their values, preferences and circumstances.

3. Assess patient capacity:
Capacity refers to the patient's ability to understand the information provided, evaluate options and make an informed decision. It is specific to each decision and may vary according to the situation. To assess capacity, we generally consider :
- The patient's understanding of the medical situation.
- Its ability to understand the consequences of different options.
- Its ability to communicate its decision.

4. Capacity dilemmas :
Sometimes patients are deemed incapable of giving

informed consent, whether due to cognitive impairment, mental illness, or other factors. In these situations :
- A legal guardian or medical representative may be asked to give consent on behalf of the patient.
- It is essential to always act in the patient's best interests, while respecting their previously expressed wishes as far as possible.

5. Informed consent in children and adolescents :
The ability of minors to give consent depends on their emotional and intellectual maturity. Although parents or guardians are generally involved, it is crucial to include the child or adolescent in discussions, depending on their level of understanding.

6. Refusal of treatment :
A capable patient has the right to refuse treatment, even if this is against medical advice. In these situations, it is vital to ensure that the patient understands the consequences of their choice.

Informed consent is not simply a formality or a signature on a document. It is a dynamic process that requires open, honest and two-way communication between the healthcare professional and the patient. By respecting patient autonomy and recognising the nuances of capacity, carers can offer care that is both ethically sound and patient-centred.

Chapter 11:
PAEDIATRIC ONCOLOGY

Key differences
between paediatric and adult cancers

Cancer is a complex disease that varies greatly according to individual and age. Paediatric cancers, although rare compared with adult cancers, have distinct features that set them apart on a number of levels. Understanding these differences is essential to ensure optimal care for each age group.

1. Types of cancer :
   - **Paediatric:** Leukaemias (particularly acute lymphoblastic leukaemia) are the most common in children. Other common cancers include brain tumours, neuroblastoma, Ewing's sarcoma and osteosarcoma.
   - **Adults:** Carcinomas (epithelial cell cancers) predominate in adults, such as lung, breast, prostate and colon cancer.
2. Causes and risk factors :
   - **Paediatric** cancers: The causes of paediatric cancers remain largely unknown. Congenital genetic mutations and certain hereditary diseases may increase the risk.
   - **Adults:** Exposure to environmental factors (tobacco, alcohol, UV radiation) and certain lifestyle habits are major causes. Family history can also play a role.
3. Growth and propagation :
   - **Paediatrics:** Childhood cancers tend to progress rapidly, but generally respond better to chemotherapy.
   - **Adults:** They may progress more slowly, but may be more resistant to certain treatments. They are also more likely to metastasise.

4. Location :
- **Paediatric:** Paediatric cancers are often found in growing parts of the body, such as bones and the central nervous system.
- **Adults:** They are often located in specific organs or tissues, such as the lungs, prostate or breast.

5. Therapeutic approach :
- **Paediatrics:** Children require specific dosages and careful monitoring of side effects. Their treatment is often centralised in specialised centres.
- **Adults:** Treatment is more varied and can be administered according to the stage of the disease, co-morbidities and the patient's age.

6. Long-term consequences :
- **Paediatrics:** Children have a longer life expectancy after treatment, but may be exposed to long-term side effects such as growth problems, fertility problems or other cancers in adulthood.
- **Adults:** Long-term consequences are generally associated with age, co-morbidities and the specific side-effects of treatment.

7. Survival rate :
- **Paediatrics:** In general, the survival rate for paediatric cancers is higher than for adults, thanks in part to a better response to treatment.
- **Adults:** Although many adult cancers have a good survival rate when detected early, others may have a less favourable prognosis due to their aggressive nature or late detection.

Although paediatric and adult cancers share the same 'cancer' name, there are significant differences in terms of type, cause, treatment and prognosis. A thorough understanding of these distinctions is essential to ensure that each patient, whatever their age, receives appropriate care.

The role of the nurse
with children and their families

In paediatrics, nurses care not only for the child, but also for his or her family. Their role extends far beyond simply administering medication or monitoring vital signs. They often become a pillar of support, a source of information and a link between the family and the medical team.

1. Assessment and clinical care :
The nurse regularly assesses the child's state of health, monitors symptoms, administers treatments and ensures that the child is as comfortable as possible.

2. Education and information:
It provides clear and understandable information about the disease, treatment and care at home. This education helps parents to better understand the situation, to actively participate in care and to make informed decisions.

3. Emotional support:
Faced with a child's illness, emotions can run high. The nurse offers emotional support to both the child and the family, helping them to deal with feelings of fear, uncertainty and sadness.

4. Advocacy for the child:
The nurse advocates for the rights of the child, ensuring that their needs are met and that their voice is heard, even if they are too young to express themselves.

5. Collaboration with the medical team :
The nurse plays a central role in the care team, communicating the concerns, observations and needs of the child and his/her family to the other health professionals.

6. Facilitating family dynamics:
By recognising that each family has its own dynamics and needs, the nurse helps to facilitate positive family interactions and support the family as a whole.

7. Transition support :
Whether it's going home from hospital or moving from one ward to another, the nurse plays a crucial role in ensuring that this transition goes as smoothly as possible.

8. Promoting autonomy :
Depending on the child's age, the nurse encourages autonomy and independence, helping the child to participate in their care and understand their illness.

9. Assistance in difficult situations:
At the most painful moments, such as the announcement of a serious diagnosis or the end of life, the nurse offers support, compassion and care to the child and his or her family.

10. Referral to resources :
The nurse may recommend support groups, therapies or other resources to help the family cope and find support beyond the hospital.

The role of the paediatric nurse is vast and multidimensional. By establishing a relationship of trust with the child and his or her family, the nurse provides continuity of care, emotional support and education, enhancing the child's overall well-being while accompanying the family through the challenges of the illness.

Specific challenges
palliative care in paediatrics

When faced with the serious illness of a child, paediatric palliative care presents particular challenges, often more poignant and complex than those encountered in adult palliative care. The aim of this care is to offer the child the highest possible quality of life, while supporting the family through a period of pain and uncertainty.

1. Facing injustice :
The imminent death or incurable illness of a child is often perceived as contrary to the natural order of things, which intensifies the feeling of injustice and powerlessness among family members and carers.

2. Delicate communication :
Explaining a serious illness or bleak prognosis to a child requires particular finesse. You have to present the facts in a way that is appropriate to their age and ability to understand, while preserving their innocence.

3. Support for parents :
Parents experience profound distress when faced with the suffering or imminent loss of their child. Helping them navigate this emotional storm while encouraging them to participate in decisions about their care is a major challenge.

4. Taking account of siblings :
Siblings may feel neglected or misunderstood. It is crucial to include them in the process, answer their questions and offer them emotional support.

5. Pain assessment :
Children, especially the very young, may find it difficult to express their pain. Proper assessment and management of their discomfort requires special attention and expertise.

6. Ethical decisions :
In some cases, difficult decisions about continuing or stopping treatment have to be made. These decisions have far-reaching consequences and require transparent and compassionate communication between the medical team and the family.

7. Preparing for the end of life :
Creating a peaceful, dignified and comfortable environment for the terminally ill child is essential. This may include rituals, the presence of loved ones or the incorporation of symbols and memories.

8. Support after the loss :
The period following a child's death is crucial. Parents and

family need support to cope with bereavement, and the medical team itself may need help to process its own emotions.

9. Specialised training :
Paediatric palliative carers need specific skills to meet the unique needs of these children and their families.

10. Limited resources:
In many healthcare systems, resources dedicated to paediatric palliative care are limited, which can restrict the options available for treatment and support.

Paediatric palliative care is a demanding and emotionally intense vocation. Despite the many challenges, the aim remains to ensure that every child receives compassionate, individualised and quality care, while supporting their family during and after this difficult time.

Chapter 12:
HOME CARE AND AMBULATORY CARE

The growing importance of care out of hospital

As healthcare systems evolve, an emerging trend is that more and more care is being delivered outside the traditional hospital setting. This transition to outpatient, ambulatory or home-based care has considerable advantages, but it also raises challenges. Let's look at the growing importance of this approach.

1. Demographics and patient needs :
With an ageing population and the growing prevalence of chronic illnesses, the demand for regular, long-term care is increasing. However, managing these illnesses in hospital over a long period is neither practical nor cost-effective.

2. Cost and effectiveness :
Providing care at home or in outpatient clinics can often be less costly than prolonged hospitalisation. This frees up hospital resources for more acute cases or those requiring specialist care.

3. Patient quality of life:
Being able to receive care in a familiar environment can improve patient well-being, reduce stress and facilitate recovery. It also avoids the risks associated with long hospital stays, such as nosocomial infections.

4. Technological advances :
Technological innovations now make it possible to monitor, diagnose and even treat patients remotely. Telemedicine, for example, makes it possible to consult specialists without the patient having to travel.

5. Continuity of care :
Outpatient care favours a holistic approach, where the

patient is seen as a whole, integrating his or her family and social environment. This encourages better coordination between healthcare professionals and a smooth transition between different levels of care.

6. Patient empowerment:

Receiving care at home or learning to manage a chronic illness outside a medical establishment encourages patient autonomy and responsibility.

7. Reducing hospital congestion:

With hospitals often overcrowded, moving certain services or treatments to outpatient clinics or at home can help relieve congestion and prioritise the most urgent cases.

8. Family support:

By avoiding lengthy hospital stays, patients can benefit from the direct support of their family and close friends, which is essential to their emotional well-being.

9. Changes in medical training:

Healthcare professionals are increasingly trained to provide care outside the hospital setting, strengthening the capacity of healthcare systems to meet this growing demand.

10. Logistical challenges :

While there are many benefits, out-of-hospital care is not without its challenges. Patient safety must be guaranteed, effective communication between carers must be ensured, and access to the necessary equipment and medicines must be guaranteed.

As the needs of the population change and technology continues to evolve, it is likely that out-of-hospital care will become increasingly important. Properly orchestrated, this transition can lead to improved quality of care, greater efficiency and a better patient experience.

Adapting protocols and practices

Medical protocols and clinical practices are the foundations of healthcare, ensuring the safety, quality and consistency of care provided to patients. However, in a constantly changing medical environment, it is essential to regularly review and adapt these protocols. Let's take a closer look at this need for adaptation and the issues surrounding it.

1. Developments in scientific knowledge :
Medical research is progressing at breakneck speed, discovering new treatments, approaches and knowledge. Protocols need to be updated to reflect these advances and ensure that patients receive the most up-to-date care.

2. Introduction of new technologies :
The advent of new technologies, such as innovative medical devices or telemedicine tools, requires appropriate training and updating of practices to ensure safe and effective use.

3. Feedback:
Feedback from healthcare professionals and patients can reveal areas for improvement in existing protocols. This valuable feedback enables practices to be fine-tuned to better meet patients' needs.

4. Demographic variability :
Populations are changing in terms of age, ethnic diversity and health needs. Protocols need to be adapted to meet the specific needs of these varied populations.

5. Economic issues :
Budgetary constraints may require adjustments to protocols to maximise the effectiveness of care while respecting financial limits.

6. Regulatory watch :
Medical laws and regulations evolve, sometimes imposing new standards or criteria that protocols must comply with.

7. Health crises:
Situations such as the COVID-19 pandemic require rapid adaptation of protocols to deal with urgent and unexpected medical issues.

8. Individualised approaches :
With the rise of personalised medicine, protocols need to be flexible enough to allow care to be tailored to each patient, while maintaining quality standards.

9. Interdisciplinary collaboration :
Modern medicine favours a collaborative approach. Protocols must therefore be designed to encourage cooperation between medical specialities.

10. Education and training:
Whenever a protocol is changed, training of healthcare professionals is crucial to ensure effective and consistent implementation.

Adapting protocols and practices is a vital part of ensuring that healthcare is relevant and effective. This requires constant monitoring, responsiveness to new developments, and a commitment to putting the patient at the heart of all decisions. In an ever-changing medical world, this flexibility and commitment to continuous improvement are more crucial than ever.

Benefits and challenges home care

As the healthcare system evolves, home care is gaining in popularity and becoming a solid alternative to traditional hospital care for many patients. This form of care has many advantages, but it also comes with its own unique challenges. Let's take a closer look at the two sides of this coin.

Advantages :

1. Patient comfort :

Patients are cared for in familiar surroundings familiar environment, which can reduce the stress and anxiety often associated with hospital stays.

2. Personalised care :

Care can be tailored to the individual needs individual needs, taking into account the patient's environment and lifestyle.

3. Cost reduction :

Home care can often cost less than hospital care than hospital care, both for patients and for healthcare and for healthcare systems.

4. Less exposure to infections :

By avoiding the hospital environment, patients can reduce their risk of hospital-acquired hospital-acquired infections.

5. Family support :

Home care allows for greater involvement of the family involvement, strengthening the patient's support support network.

6. Continuity of care :

Home care can provide a smoother transition between hospitalisation and a return to normal life, ensuring life, ensuring continuity of care.

Challenges :

1. Access to equipment and technologies :

The patient's home may not be equipped with the advanced advanced medical technologies available hospital.

2. Medical surveillance :

Outside a hospital environment, it can be difficult to difficult to provide constant medical supervision monitoring.

3. Training and skills :

Not all healthcare professionals are necessarily
trained or comfortable providing care in the
home. home care.

4. Communication :

Coordination between the various parties involved
(doctors, nurses, therapists) can be more
complicated at home complicated at home than in hospital.

5. Medical emergencies :

In the event of a complication or emergency, the
time to transport a patient from home to hospital can
from home to hospital can be a problem.

6. Safety :

Healthcare professionals can face   s e c u r i t y
challenges when they visit unknown homes.
unknown homes.

7. Isolation :

Although the home is comfortable, some
patients may feel isolated if they do not receive
regular   without regular visits from family or
friends.   family or friends.

Home care offers a fantastic opportunity to improve the
quality of care while meeting patients' individual needs.
However, to maximise its effectiveness and minimise risks,
it is essential to approach this care with careful planning
and appropriate training.

Chapter 13:
CULTURAL DIVERSITY IN ONCOLOGY

Understanding cultural differences and their impact on care

In today's globalised world, cultural diversity is an increasingly frequent guest in healthcare establishments. This mosaic of traditions, beliefs and practices has a profound influence on the way people approach illness, healing and, more generally, their interactions with healthcare professionals. Understanding these nuances is crucial if we are to offer high-quality, appropriate care that respects each patient.

Each culture has its own beliefs about what causes illness, how it should be treated, and who should be involved in the care process. For example, in some cultures, illness may be seen as divine punishment or the result of an energy imbalance. Elsewhere, traditional remedies or spiritual rituals may be used to complement, or even replace, conventional medical treatments.

Cultural differences can also influence how pain and suffering are perceived, how they are expressed and how they should be managed. While some will see open expression of pain as a sign of weakness, others will see it as a legitimate way of seeking help or attention.

These differences also extend to interpersonal relationships and expectations about the role of carers. In some cultures, the doctor is seen as an unquestioned authority, while in others he or she is seen more as a partner in the care process. Similarly, issues such as eye contact, physical proximity and the way questions are asked can be perceived very differently in different cultural contexts.

Failure to take account of these cultural variations can lead to misunderstandings, loss of trust or less effective care. Patients may feel misunderstood, devalued or even stigmatised. In the worst cases, they may even give up on vital treatment.

But recognising cultural diversity is not just about avoiding mistakes. It is also a tremendous opportunity. By integrating this diversity into their approach to care, healthcare professionals can establish a deeper and more meaningful relationship with their patients, fostering greater cooperation and better adherence to the treatments offered. Listening, continuous training and curiosity are all tools for developing solid cultural competence.

The richness of different cultures is a treasure that healthcare professionals must cherish and understand. It is by fully embracing this diversity that we can offer truly holistic, respectful and personalised care.

Adapting communication and actions to take account of diversity

At the heart of the therapeutic relationship is communication, the cornerstone of effective care and patient satisfaction. In an increasingly cosmopolitan environment, the art of communicating with patients from different cultures, backgrounds and beliefs is becoming crucial. Knowing how to adapt one's communication and interventions to this cultural diversity is not only an essential skill, but also a profound sign of respect for each patient.

Firstly, it is essential to recognise that each individual has a unique set of beliefs, values and experiences. Even within the same culture, there can be significant variations. So a stereotyped or generalised approach should be avoided. Instead, adopt an attitude of continuous learning, active listening and open-mindedness.

The first step towards appropriate communication is self-reflection. It is essential that healthcare professionals take the time to recognise their own prejudices, values and beliefs in order to avoid unintentional projections onto the patient. It is also beneficial to receive regular training in cultural competence, keeping abreast of the nuances and subtleties specific to each culture.

Another crucial aspect is language skills. When the patient is not fluent in the language of the carer, the use of professional interpreters can be invaluable. It's not just a question of translating words, but also nuances, emotions and intentions. This ensures that the patient fully understands the information and recommendations, while feeling heard and respected.

When carrying out medical procedures, it is essential to take account of the patient's cultural beliefs. For example, some cultures may have reservations about certain surgical procedures or blood transfusions. In such cases, an open and respectful discussion with the patient and his or her family can often lead to a compromise or an alternative acceptable to all parties.

Rituals and cultural practices can also influence how a patient wishes to receive care. Some may prefer prayers or rituals before an operation, while others may have specific dietary preferences. Taking these elements into account and incorporating them as far as possible into the care plan builds trust and patient acceptance.

Adapting communication and interventions to cultural diversity is a journey, an ongoing exploration of the depths of humanity. It is a commitment to excellence in care, a promise to see each patient not as a box to be ticked, but as a unique individual, with his or her own needs, aspirations and stories.

Resources and training
for care culturally competent

In the vast world of healthcare, culturally competent care is fast becoming a necessity. Clinicians who understand and respect the cultural beliefs, values and traditions of their patients are better equipped to provide quality care and build trusting relationships. Fortunately, there are many resources and training courses designed to reinforce this essential skill. Let's take a look at some of these avenues for culturally sensitive care.

- Specialised   training in cultural skills :
    - Many institutes and universities offer modules or programmes dedicated to training in cultural competence. These courses generally aim to provide healthcare professionals with the tools to identify and overcome cultural barriers, as well as to develop effective communication with patients from diverse backgrounds.
- Seminars and workshops :
    - Taking part in workshops or seminars organised by professional associations or specialist groups can be an excellent way of acquiring practical knowledge on specific subjects related to cultural diversity.
- Guides and manuals :
    - There are many manuals that provide detailed overviews of different cultures, their health beliefs, practices and expectations of carers. These resources are invaluable in anticipating

and understanding the specific needs of each cultural group.

- Mentoring programmes :
  - Finding a mentor with expertise in cultural competence can offer personalised learning. Mentoring allows a direct exchange of experiences, challenges and solutions in culturally competent care.
- Online resources :
  - With the proliferation of digital technologies, many online training modules are now available. These e-learning courses often offer flexibility, enabling professionals to learn at their own pace.
- Networks and associations :
  - Joining associations dedicated to multicultural health or networks of professionals with heightened cultural sensitivity can be beneficial. These platforms encourage the sharing of information, strategies and best practice.
- Intercultural exchanges :
  - Exchange programmes can offer direct immersion in another culture, enabling a deep understanding and appreciation of cultural nuances.
- Interaction with local communities :
  - Taking part in community events, discussion groups or forums allows you to connect directly with various cultural groups, listen to their concerns and understand their needs.

The quest for culturally competent care is an ongoing commitment. It requires an open mind, a willingness to learn and a passion for offering the best possible care to every patient, whatever their cultural heritage. With the resources and training available, healthcare professionals can equip and enrich their practices to meet the needs of everyone in our diverse world.

Chapter 14:
TRAINING AND MENTORING

Career development paths in oncology

The specialty of oncology offers a wealth of opportunities for healthcare professionals wishing to develop their careers. As a dynamic and constantly evolving discipline, oncology not only offers the opportunity to develop knowledge and clinical skills, but also to explore a variety of roles and responsibilities depending on individual aspirations. Here's an overview of the different career paths available in oncology:

- Specialisation in oncology subfield :
    - **Medical oncology**: focused on chemotherapy and other drug treatments.
    - **Surgical oncology**: focused on surgical interventions to remove tumours.
    - **Radiological oncology or radiotherapy**: specialising in the treatment of cancer using radiation.
    - **Paediatric oncology: treatment of** cancers in children and adolescents.
- Clinical nurse specialising in oncology :
    - With further training, a nurse can become a specialist clinical nurse, playing a crucial role in the assessment, planning and implementation of oncology care.

- Oncology research :
    - For those with a passion for science and innovation, a career in cancer research may be an option. This may involve clinical studies, translational research or basic research.
- Management and administration :

- • The roles of manager or administrator in oncology involve supervising operations, managing human resources and ensuring the quality of care.
- • Education and training :
  - • Becoming an oncology educator or trainer enables you to train the next generation of healthcare professionals, whether through continuing education, seminars or within academic institutions.
- • Genetic counselling in oncology :
  - • With the rise of personalised medicine, genetic counsellors play a key role in identifying genetic risks for cancer and advising patients and their families.
- • Palliative and supportive care :
  - • This specialisation focuses on patients' quality of life, treating the pain, symptoms and stress of cancer.
- • Psycho-oncology :
  - • Psycho-oncology focuses on the psychological aspects of cancer, offering emotional support and therapeutic interventions to patients and their families.
- • Oncology pharmacy :
  - • Pharmacists specialising in oncology play an essential role in managing medicines, advising on drug interactions and educating patients.
- • Consultation and advocacy :
  - • Some professionals choose to become consultants, advising on specific aspects of oncology, or patient advocates, working to improve cancer policy and practice.

As a medical field, oncology offers an impressive range of opportunities for professionals who want to broaden their horizons, deepen their skills and make a significant difference to the lives of their patients. Each path offers its own challenges and rewards, but all are united by a common goal: to improve cancer care and the quality of life of patients.

The importance of mentoring for new professionals

The transition from student to professional is a fascinating journey, often fraught with uncertainty, discovery and unexpected challenges. For new professionals in any discipline, the transition can be both exhilarating and disconcerting. This is where the invaluable role of mentoring comes in, providing a compass for those venturing into the vast professional world.

At the heart of mentoring is the relationship between mentor and mentee. It's a dynamic relationship based on trust, guidance and shared experience. The mentor, often an experienced professional, offers not only technical knowledge, but also sound advice, practical tips and, above all, a perspective based on years of practice and experience.

The importance of mentoring rests on several essential pillars:
- **Accelerated learning**: With mentoring, new professionals can avoid common mistakes, understand the nuances of their job more quickly and adopt best practice from the outset. It's less about reinventing the wheel and more about leveraging accumulated experience to make effective progress.
- **Confidence-building**: Venturing into an unfamiliar field can give rise to doubts and uncertainties. The support of a mentor reassures the mentee, encouraging them to take initiative, ask questions and develop their professional confidence.

- **Professional network**: A good mentor can also introduce the mentee to a professional network, opening doors to opportunities, collaborations and career advancement.
- **Personal development**: In addition to professional skills, mentoring can also play a key role in the mentee's personal development. This may involve learning how to manage stress, balance work and personal life, or develop leadership skills.
- **Constructive feedback**: One of the most valuable aspects of mentoring is the mentor's ability to provide honest and caring feedback, helping the mentee to identify their strengths and areas for improvement.
- **Continuity of skills**: Mentoring also ensures that skills and knowledge are passed on from one generation to the next, guaranteeing the continuity and evolution of professional know-how.

Mentoring is much more than just professional guidance. It's a rewarding partnership that shapes, inspires and propels new professionals to heights they might otherwise have thought unattainable. By investing in mentoring, we are investing not only in the future of an individual, but also in the longevity and excellence of an entire profession.

Continuing training and opportunities for specialisation

In the ever-changing world of health, technology and science, keeping up to date is not only essential for professional competence, it is also an ethical imperative. Continuing education and specialisation opportunities play a central role in meeting this need.

Continuing education is much more than simply updating your knowledge. It represents a commitment to excellence, a thirst for continuous improvement and a recognition that learning never stops, regardless of seniority or expertise in a given field. It offers professionals :

- **Updating skills**: With technological advances, new research and regulatory changes, it's essential to regularly update your skills to provide the best possible care and service.
- **Vocational rehabilitation**: Continuing training enables professionals to adjust or redirect their career path in response to changing market needs or personal interests.
- **Networking**: Taking part in training courses, seminars or workshops is also a valuable opportunity to network, exchange ideas and collaborate with peers and experts from different backgrounds.
- **Accreditation and certification**: In many fields, continuing education is a requirement for maintaining accreditation, licensing or certification, thus ensuring credibility and professional recognition.

Specialisation opportunities, on the other hand, enable professionals to deepen their skills in specific niches or areas of interest. This has a number of advantages:
- **In-depth expertise**: Specialising allows you to acquire in-depth expertise, which can lead to recognition as an expert in the field.
- **Career opportunities**: Specialists are often sought after for specific positions, consultancies or leadership roles.
- **Significant contributions**: With a specialisation, professionals can make a significant contribution to the advancement of their field, whether through research, innovation or education.

Finally, it should be stressed that continuing education and specialisation are not linear paths. Training opportunities can inspire new specialisations, and vice versa. It's a journey of continuous learning that reflects passion, dedication and commitment to excellence. In a fast-changing world, embracing continuing education and specialisation opportunities is not just a necessity, but a privilege that enriches careers, professionalism and, ultimately, the quality of services offered to society.

Chapter 15:
LOGISTICAL CHALLENGES
AND ORGANISATIONAL

Managing schedules and patient flows

In the medical field, and particularly in oncology, effective management of patient schedules and flows is crucial to ensuring optimal care delivery. It influences not only patient satisfaction and well-being, but also the productivity of the care team. Achieving this often delicate balance requires a structured, flexible and patient-centred approach.

Planning, as such, is like a complex choreography. It takes into account :
- **Forecasting**: Analysing historical data to anticipate inflows, taking into account seasonal variations, days of the week and possible epidemics or emergencies.
- **Flexibility**: rapidly adapt resources, whether in terms of staff, available rooms or equipment, to meet changing needs.
- **Prioritisation**: Identifying which patients need urgent treatment and which can wait, without compromising the quality of care.

Patient flow, on the other hand, refers to the way in which patients move through the various stages of their care. Effective management involves :
- **Reception**: Ensuring a warm and informative welcome on arrival, reducing patient stress and facilitating the first stage of their care.
- **Guidance**: Directing patients efficiently to the right units or specialists to minimise waiting times.

- **Coordination**: Ensuring that all the professionals involved in a patient's care - nurses, doctors, technicians, etc. - are informed and synchronised.
- **Follow-up**: Ensuring that each patient receives the information they need for the next steps, whether it's another appointment, hospitalisation or follow-up at home.

In addition, **modern technologies** such as electronic appointment management systems and telecommunications applications can help optimise these processes, offering greater visibility and flexibility.

However, it is fundamental to remember that behind every appointment, every schedule and every flow, there is a patient - a person with concerns, hopes and needs. The key to successful management lies in balancing operational efficiency with compassion, ensuring that each patient is treated not just as a number, but as a unique individual deserving of respect, attention and quality care.

Technological innovations in the management of oncology departments

Technology is advancing at breakneck speed, and the medical sector, particularly oncology, is no exception to this revolution. These advances are not just limited to treatments, but are also transforming the way in which oncology services are managed, creating better co-ordination, efficiency and improved care for patients.

- **Electronic medical records (EMR)**: The move from paper records to electronic systems has facilitated rapid access to patient information, exchanges between specialists and continuous updating. They enable coordinated, personalised care, avoiding duplication of tests and drug interactions.

- **Telemedicine**: Thanks to virtual consultations, patients can benefit from the expertise of specialists, even if they are geographically distant. This is particularly beneficial for those living in rural areas or who have difficulty travelling.
- **Advanced medical imaging**: Innovations such as positron emission tomography (PET) and multiparametric magnetic resonance provide more precise images, facilitating early detection and monitoring of tumours.
- **Artificial Intelligence (AI)**: AI can help rapidly analyse large volumes of data, facilitating diagnosis, risk prediction and even treatment planning. Algorithms can detect nuances in medical images that are often invisible to the naked eye.
- **Wearable technologies and healthcare applications**: Connected watches, bracelets and other devices can monitor parameters such as heart rate, oxygen levels in the blood and temperature in real time. This data, transmitted to healthcare professionals, can help anticipate and manage complications.
- **Integrated care management platforms**: These systems facilitate communication between all those involved in an oncology care pathway - surgeons, oncologists, radiologists, nurses, etc. - ensuring comprehensive, coordinated care. - to ensure comprehensive, coordinated care.
- **Planning and simulation systems**: In fields such as radiotherapy, advanced software is used to simulate treatment to optimise the dose delivered to the tumour while sparing healthy tissue.
- **Virtual training and simulations**: Virtual and augmented reality offer professionals platforms for

training, simulating operations or technical gestures, and familiarising themselves with complex situations without risk to the patient.

Despite all these technological advances, it is essential to bear in mind that technology is a tool at the service of people. It must be used ethically, ensuring data protection and keeping the patient at the heart of all decisions. The combination of human skills and technological innovation is the key to shaping the future of oncology.

Coordination with other departments and medical specialities

The complex, multi-dimensional nature of oncology requires close collaboration with a variety of medical departments and specialities. This interaction ensures that patients receive comprehensive care that meets both their medical needs and their quality of life.

- **Surgery**: Cancer treatment often requires surgery to remove a tumour. Close collaboration with the surgery department ensures a smooth transition from diagnosis to operation, and then to recovery and post-operative care.
- **Radiology**: Radiologists play a central role in diagnosing and monitoring tumours and planning treatment. Medical imaging is used to assess the size, location and evolution of tumours.
- **Haematology**: For blood cancers such as leukaemia or lymphoma, interaction with haematologists is essential in developing and monitoring treatment protocols.
- **Pathology**: Pathologists analyse tissue samples to confirm the malignant nature of cells and define the

exact type of cancer, information that is crucial in determining the appropriate treatment.

- **Pharmacy**: Working with pharmacists ensures that medicines, particularly chemotherapeutic agents, are administered correctly, monitoring drug interactions and managing side effects.
- **Palliative care**: When cancer is at an advanced stage, the focus is on relieving symptoms and improving quality of life, requiring close collaboration with palliative care teams.
- **Psychology and psychiatry**: The fight against cancer is as much mental as it is physical. Psychologists and psychiatrists provide emotional support to patients and their families, helping them to manage the anxiety, depression and stress associated with the disease.
- **Nutrition**: Nutrition plays a key role in the well-being of cancer patients. Working with nutritionists helps address common dietary challenges, such as loss of appetite or nausea.
- **Physiotherapy and rehabilitation**: After surgery or major treatment, patients may need rehabilitation to regain their mobility or functionality, making collaboration with physiotherapists essential.
- **Social services**: Supporting patients and their families with non-medical challenges such as logistics, finances and access to care.
- **Other specialities**: Depending on the type and location of the cancer, other specialists may be involved, such as gastroenterologists, lung specialists, endocrinologists, etc.

Coordination between these different services requires open channels of communication, regular multidisciplinary conferences and shared medical records. It is this integrated and holistic approach that ensures that every patient receives the best possible care, tailored to their specific needs.

Chapter 16:
THE IMPACT OF TECHNOLOGY IN ONCOLOGY

The emergence of telemedicine and its implications

Telemedicine is a revolution in the way medical care is delivered, using information and communication technologies to provide remote consultations, often in real time. In oncology, as in many other areas of medicine, telemedicine offers a multitude of advantages, but also poses certain challenges.

- **Improved access to care**: Telemedicine enables patients living in remote areas, where access to oncology specialists may be limited, to receive high-quality consultations and follow-up care without having to travel long distances. This reduces costs, travel time and the stress associated with medical visits.
- **Real-time monitoring**: Technologies enable continuous monitoring of patients, particularly those receiving treatment at home. Connected devices can transmit vital data, enabling healthcare professionals to act quickly in the event of a problem.
- **Savings for the healthcare system**: By reducing the need for face-to-face appointments, the costs associated with hospital visits are reduced. In addition, early management of complications using telemedicine can prevent costly hospitalisations.
- **Training and mentoring**: Healthcare professionals can benefit from remote training sessions, webinars and mentoring, giving them greater access to expertise and educational resources.

- **Technological challenges**: Although telemedicine offers many benefits, it also requires a robust technological infrastructure. Rural or underdeveloped areas may not have adequate connectivity, limiting the benefits of telemedicine.
- **Confidentiality issues**: Transmitting sensitive medical data via the Internet poses security and confidentiality challenges. It is imperative to ensure that patient information is protected against data breaches.
- **Interpersonal complexities**: Face-to-face contact plays a crucial role in establishing trust between patient and healthcare professional. Telemedicine can make this relationship less personal, which can affect the quality of communication.
- **Regulatory developments**: With the rise of telemedicine, many countries and regions have had to adapt or create regulations to govern this new form of healthcare provision. This includes the legitimacy of remote consultations, insurance coverage and licensing issues for doctors practising across borders.
- **Integration into workflows**: Integrating telemedicine into existing hospital workflows requires training and adjustment for both healthcare professionals and patients.

The emergence of telemedicine in oncology presents an exciting opportunity to improve access to care and modernise patient management. However, it is essential to navigate carefully, ensuring that the quality of care is maintained and that the challenges are addressed.

Technological tools at the patient's service

The digital age has brought a wave of innovations in the medical field, making patient care more efficient, personalised and accessible. In oncology, these advances are having a considerable impact, not only in terms of diagnosis and treatment, but also in the way patients experience their medical journey. Let's take a look at how these technological tools are serving oncology patients today:

- **Dedicated mobile applications**: Numerous applications have been developed to help patients monitor their treatment, manage their medical appointments, record their symptoms or even obtain information about their condition. These applications often offer reminders to take medication, advice on managing side effects and a space to note down questions to ask during consultations.
- **Patient portals**: These online platforms allow patients to access their medical records, communicate directly with their healthcare teams, consult their test results and schedule appointments. This gives patients a greater sense of autonomy and control.
- **Connected devices**: Whether monitoring vital signs, glucose levels or other parameters, wearables and other connected devices offer real-time monitoring, enabling us to anticipate and react quickly in the event of complications.
- **Virtual reality**: Used in some centres, virtual reality can help distract patients during long or uncomfortable treatments. It can also be a therapeutic tool, for example to manage anxiety or pain.

- **Telemedicine**: As mentioned above, telemedicine allows remote consultations, which is particularly beneficial for those living far from specialist centres.
- **Artificial Intelligence (AI)**: AI is increasingly used to help interpret medical images, improving the accuracy of diagnosis. It can also help personalise treatments by predicting a patient's response to a specific therapy.
- **Medical chatbots**: These virtual assistants can answer frequently asked questions, guide patients through the stages of treatment or even provide advice on managing side effects.
- **3D printing**: Whether to create custom-made prostheses or to model a tumour in 3D before surgery, 3D printing has found numerous applications in oncology.
- **Education and support platforms**: Numerous dedicated websites and forums offer patients a wealth of information as well as a supportive community where they can share their experiences and receive advice.

The integration of these technologies into the oncology patient care pathway has not only improved the quality and efficiency of care, but has also strengthened the patient's active role in their own care. However, it is crucial to ensure that these tools are used ethically and safely, always putting the patient's best interests first.

Future prospects : artificial intelligence, virtual reality and other innovations

In the constantly evolving world of medicine, and more specifically in oncology, technological innovations play a decisive role. These advances promise to redefine the way care is delivered, personalise treatments and improve patients' quality of life. Let's take a closer look at some of these prospects for the future, which are already shaping the face of modern oncology.

- Artificial intelligence (AI) in oncology:
    - **Early diagnosis**: Thanks to AI, the ability to detect cancers at an early stage could increase significantly. Algorithms can analyse medical images with extreme accuracy, often surpassing that of humans.
    - **Predicting disease progression**: AI can help model how a specific cancer might progress, enabling earlier interventions.
    - **Personalised treatment**: AI-based systems could predict how a specific patient will respond to a treatment, enabling truly individualised care.
- Virtual and augmented reality:
    - **Medical training**: Surgeons can carry out complex oncology operations in a virtual environment before performing them on real patients.
    - **Pain and anxiety management**: Immersive experiences can help divert patients' attention from pain or stress during invasive procedures or treatments.
- Gene therapies and personalised therapies :
    - By understanding the genome of a patient or tumour, it is possible to develop tailor-made treatments that specifically target the genetic abnormalities responsible for cancer.
- Nano-medicine :
    - Nanoparticles can be used to target and deliver drugs directly into cancer cells, reducing side effects on healthy cells.

- Robotics in surgery :
  - Assisted robots can perform surgery with greater precision, minimising damage to healthy tissue and speeding up recovery.
- Bioprinting :
  - The use of 3D printing to create biological tissue has the potential to revolutionise grafting and post-operative reconstruction in oncology.
- Connected patient monitoring platforms :
  - Wearable devices can continuously monitor vital signs and other indicators, enabling early intervention in the event of complications.
- Advanced telemedicine :
  - In addition to remote consultations, telemedicine could include remotely-assisted procedures, where a specialist guides a local health professional through interventions.

Each of these innovations promises to transform oncology, offering renewed hope and a better quality of life for patients. However, it is essential to approach these advances with caution, ensuring that medical ethics are upheld and that access to new technologies is equitable for all patients, whatever their circumstances.

Chapter 17:
FUTURE PROSPECTS

Innovations in oncology:
what the future holds

Oncology, the medical discipline devoted to the prevention, diagnosis, treatment and monitoring of cancer, is undergoing a major revolution thanks to technological and scientific innovations. These advances are pushing back the boundaries of what we thought possible, and offering renewed hope to millions of patients around the world. Let's take a look at the main innovations that could define the future of oncology.

- Immunotherapy and targeted therapies:
    - Targeted therapies, which target specific genetic mutations in cancer cells, offer more precise treatments with fewer side effects. In addition, immunotherapy, which boosts the patient's own immune system to fight the cancer, has shown promising results, particularly for traditionally resistant cancers.
- Genome sequencing and personalised medicine:
    - Genomic sequencing makes it possible to identify the specific mutations present in each tumour, leading to tailor-made treatments designed for each patient. This ultra-personalised approach should increase the chances of successful treatment.
- Virtual reality (VR) and augmented reality (AR):
    - These technologies can improve surgeon training and help plan complex operations. In addition, they offer tools for managing patients' pain and anxiety, immersing them in soothing environments during treatment.

110

- Artificial Intelligence (AI) and Machine Learning:
    - AI can analyse huge datasets to identify patterns that would be impossible for a human to detect. This can improve diagnosis, predict disease progression and personalise treatments.
- Gene therapies and CRISPR :
    - Therapies that directly target the DNA or RNA of cancer cells, thanks in particular to gene-editing technologies such as CRISPR, could offer cures for certain types of cancer.
- Microbiome and cancer :
    - The growing understanding of the role of the microbiome (all the micro-organisms present in our body) in health and disease could lead to therapeutic approaches that modify this microbiome to fight cancer.
- Nano-medicine :
    - Nanoparticles can target and deliver drugs directly to cancer cells, offering unrivalled precision and reducing side effects.
- Combinatorial therapies :
    - By using several treatments in tandem, doctors can increase overall effectiveness and reduce the chance of the cancer developing resistance.
- Innovations in radiotherapy :
    - New techniques, such as proton therapy, target tumours with greater precision, minimising damage to surrounding healthy tissue.
- Connectivity and remote care :
    - Telemedicine, combined with connected patient monitoring devices, could enable constant monitoring and rapid intervention, while offering care in the comfort of the patient's own home.

These and other innovations promise a bright future for oncology. The major challenge will be to ensure that these advances are accessible to everyone, regardless of their geographical or socio-economic situation, and that they are integrated into the treatment process in an ethical and patient-centred way.

The role of the nurse in clinical research

At the heart of the evolution of medical care, at the frontier between science and compassion, lies clinical research, a field in which nurses have gradually carved out an undeniable and fundamental place. Historically seen as a profession devoted primarily to direct care, nursing has spread its wings to embrace the challenges and potential of clinical research, reinforcing its multifaceted role in the medical panorama.

In direct contact with patients, nurses are often the face of clinical research. They are the ones who explain, reassure and support patients at every stage of a clinical trial. This proximity to the patient gives nurses a unique perspective that is crucial to the proper and ethical implementation of studies. It's not just a question of administering a treatment or following a protocol to the letter, but of understanding and anticipating patients' needs and reactions, and guaranteeing their comfort and safety.

But the research nurse's mission doesn't stop there. As well as administering care, they play a key role in data collection, ensuring that every piece of information is accurate, relevant and reliable. This reliability is essential, because it is on this data that future medical advances are based. Their meticulous observations, their detailed notes, are the cornerstones of discoveries that will improve care for future generations.

Clinical research is also fraught with ethical challenges. And once again, nurses are on the front line. In their role as defenders of the patient's interests, they must ensure that consent is not only informed, but freely given. They ensure that each patient is treated with dignity, respect and understanding, thereby guaranteeing the integrity of the entire research process.

Finally, nurses actively contribute to the design and improvement of research protocols. Their day-to-day practical experience, intuition and nursing know-how can suggest adjustments or innovative approaches that make research more effective or more humane.

It is this confluence of skills, compassion and curiosity that makes nurses an essential pillar of clinical research. By embracing this facet of their profession, nurses continue to prove that their role goes far beyond direct care, extending to the very heart of medical innovation.

Continuing professional development

In the dynamic and ever-changing world of medicine, where new discoveries, techniques and approaches are emerging every day, continuing professional development (CPD) is not just a choice, but an imperative necessity. For oncology nurses, as for all healthcare professionals, CPD is the guarantee of a practice that is up to date, relevant and focused on patient safety and well-being.

CPD is a commitment, a promise made not only to oneself as a professional, but also to patients, colleagues and society as a whole. It is a commitment to never stop learning, adapting and improving, regardless of seniority or experience.

The CPD process encompasses much more than simply acquiring new skills or knowledge. It is a holistic approach that aims to improve skills, attitudes and behaviours. This includes attending training courses, reading relevant articles and publications, attending conferences, but also sharing knowledge with peers, reflecting on personal practice and adapting accordingly.

For oncology nurses, there are many advantages to CPD:

- **Improved patient care:** By keeping abreast of the latest advances and recommendations, nurses can offer cutting-edge care based on the latest evidence, ensuring the best possible outcomes for their patients.
- **Professional fulfilment:** Mastering new skills, techniques or knowledge boosts confidence and job satisfaction, helping to prevent burnout.
- **Interdisciplinary collaboration:** By sharing their knowledge and learning from other specialities, nurses strengthen interprofessional links, encouraging a collaborative approach to care.
- **Professional recognition:** Demonstrating a commitment to CPD can open the door to new career opportunities, whether in leadership, teaching or research.
- **Adaptability:** In a medical environment that is changing at breakneck speed, being proactive in your professional development ensures that you are better prepared for the changes and challenges ahead.

Continuing professional development is more than just a journey; it's a state of mind. For committed nurses, it's a pact renewed every day to offer the best of themselves, in the service of their patients and their vocation.

Chapter 18:
RESOURCES AND REFERENCES

Organisations
and professional associations

In the complex world of medicine, and particularly in the field of oncology, professional organisations and associations play a major role. These bodies provide support, resources and representation for their members, acting as beacons in the often tumultuous landscape of healthcare.

Professional organisations vary in scope, with some having an international reach and others focusing on national, regional or even speciality-specific issues. But whatever their size or field of action, they share common objectives:

- **Training and education:** They offer continuing education opportunities, workshops, conferences and symposia to help their members stay up to date in their field.
- **Research:** Many of them support or directly conduct studies and research to advance the field of oncology.
- **Advocacy:** These organisations represent their members before legislative and government bodies and decision-makers, advocating favourable policies and defending the rights and interests of healthcare professionals and patients.
- **Networking:** They provide platforms where professionals can exchange, collaborate and share their experience and knowledge.

- **Resources:** Practice guides, articles, newsletters and other materials are often made available to support members in their day-to-day practice.
- **Recognition:** These associations may offer certifications or distinctions, recognising excellence and expertise within the profession.

Some emblematic organisations and associations in the field of oncology could include:
- The European Organisation for Research and Treatment of Cancer (EORTC)
- The American Society of Clinical Oncology (ASCO)
- The French Oncology Society (SFO)
- The International Society of Nurses in Cancer Care (ISNCC)

For the oncology nurse, becoming actively involved in these organisations can offer a multitude of benefits, from professional enrichment to the creation of lasting links with colleagues from all over the world. By bringing individuals together around a common goal, these associations strengthen the profession as a whole, contributing to the continuous improvement of oncology care.

Recommended books and publications

For any healthcare professional working in the complex world of oncology, specialist literature is an invaluable resource. It offers in-depth knowledge, practical case studies, recent discoveries and much other essential information. Here is a selection of books and publications particularly recommended for oncology nurses:

Fundamental works :
- **"Oncology for the nurse"** by Jeanne Phillips: A comprehensive handbook covering the fundamentals

of oncology care, from the biological basis of cancer to treatment approaches.

- **"Guide pratique de l'infirmière en oncologie"** by Laura Ollier: A must-have resource covering the specifics of the nursing role in the care of cancer patients.
- **"Pain management in oncology"** by Marie-Claire Groheux: This book looks at strategies for assessing and managing pain in oncology patients.

Trade journals :

- **"Journal of Clinical Oncology**: Published by the American Society of Clinical Oncology, this journal is a major source of research articles, reviews and commentaries in the field of oncology.
- **"Cancer Nursing Practice"**: Focusing on oncology nursing practice, this journal addresses the challenges and issues facing the profession, while offering case studies and innovative approaches.

Resources on communication and ethics :

- **"Difficult Conversations in Medicine"** by Elaine Stavert: A guide to navigating delicate discussions with patients and their families, from diagnostic announcements to end-of-life care planning.
- **"Ethics in Oncology: A Practical Approach"** by Isabelle Martel: This book looks at the ethical dilemmas commonly encountered in oncology and suggests strategies for dealing with them.

Innovation resources :

- **"Technology and innovation in oncology"** by Sylvain Delafontaine: An exploration of recent technological advances in oncology and their impact on clinical practice.

Practical guides :

- **"Pharmacology in oncology: a guide for nurses"** by Corinne Bruna: A reference book on the drugs used in oncology, their mechanisms of action, side effects and administration.

- **"Soins palliatifs en oncologie : approche infirmière"** by Claire Deschamps: A comprehensive guide to caring for terminally ill patients, focusing on comfort, dignity and support.

Each book or publication on this list is a goldmine of information, advice and expertise. Together, they provide a comprehensive overview of oncology, arming nurses with the knowledge and skills they need to provide the best possible care for their patients.

Web sources for continuous updating

With the rapid evolution of oncology treatments and protocols, it is crucial for nurses and other healthcare professionals to stay informed. Web sources are an effective way of accessing the latest news, research and recommendations. Here is a list of trusted web sources for ongoing oncology updates:

- Professional organisations and research institutes :
    - American Society of Clinical Oncology (ASCO): www.asco.org
    - A leading organisation that regularly publishes recommendations, guidelines and updates on oncology treatments.
    - World Health Organization (WHO) - Cancer section : www.who.int
    - Information on cancer prevalence, global policies and care guidelines.
    - French National Cancer Institute (INCa): www.e-cancer.fr
    - Provides resources, studies and news on cancer in France.

- Professional forums and communities :
    - Oncology Nursing Society (ONS) : www.ons.org
    - A platform dedicated to oncology nurses offering training, news and a forum for exchanging ideas with peers.
    - **Cancer Care**: www.cancercare.org
    - Offers webinars, training and resources for professionals.
- Journal and research portals :
    - **PubMed** : www.ncbi.nlm.nih.gov/pubmed
    - A key database for scientific articles in medicine, with a section dedicated to oncology.
    - **ClinicalTrials.gov** : www.clinicaltrials.gov
    - Follow the latest clinical trials in oncology.
- Resources for patients and the general public :
    - **Cancer.Net**: www.cancer.net
    - Provides cancer information, news and resources for patients and their families, but is also useful for professionals.
- Pharmaceutical databases :
    - **Medscape Oncology** : www.medscape.com/oncology
    - Medical news, articles and pharmacological resources dedicated to oncology.
- Technology and innovation :
    - **Oncology Times**: www.oncology-times.com
    - Highlights the latest innovations, research and news in oncology.

Regular browsing of these sites and subscribing to their newsletters or alerts will enable nurses and healthcare professionals to keep up to date with current advances, discoveries and debates in the field of oncology.

- Professional organisations and research centres :
    - French National Cancer Institute (INCa): www.e-cancer.fr
        - A key reference point for information, research and news on cancer in France.
    - ARC Foundation for Cancer Research: www.fondation-arc.org
        - This foundation provides information on the latest advances in cancer research.
    - Société Francophone d'Onco-Gériatrie (SFOG): www.sfog.fr
        - An organisation dedicated to onco-geriatrics, combining care for the elderly and cancer treatment.
- Journal and research portals :
    - **Oncology**: www.jle.com/fr/revues/onc/
    - A medical journal focusing on oncology, with a wide range of articles and studies.
    - **Cancer information** : www.info-cancer.ca
    - A wealth of information on different types of cancer, treatments and related news.
- Professional forums and communities :
    - **OncoSuisse** : www.oncosuisse.ch
    - A Swiss platform dedicated to oncology professionals. It offers training, news and a forum for exchange.

- Resources for patients and the general public :
  - Ligue Contre le Cancer : www.ligue-cancer.net
  - It offers a wide range of information for patients, but is also useful for professionals thanks to its news and varied resources.
- Pharmaceutical databases and news :
  - **CancerOuvert** : www.cancerouvert.fr
  - A database of news and information dedicated to oncology. It focuses on new therapies.
- Professional networks :
  - Association Francophone des Soins Oncologiques de Support (AFSOS): www.afsos.org
  - This association focuses on supportive care in oncology and offers training, recommendations and news.

These resources are essential for any professional wishing to keep abreast of advances in oncology in the French-speaking world. We recommend consulting them regularly and subscribing to their newsletters or alerts to make sure you don't miss anything.